FREE FOR LIFE

FREE
FOR LIFE

A NAVY SEAL'S PATH TO INNER
FREEDOM AND OUTER PEACE

CHRISTOPHER
LEE MAHER

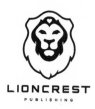

LIONCREST
PUBLISHING

FREE FOR LIFE

A Navy SEAL's Path to Inner Freedom and Outer Peace

ISBN   978-1-5445-0471-1 *Paperback*

      978-1-5445-0472-8 *Ebook*

CONTENTS

PROLOGUE

PREPARE YOURSELF

A strong, sobering message lives in the following pages.

It's not meant to make you feel comfortable.

It is meant to push you towards your edges and get you into reality.

If any part of the book bothers you, that's a good sign. Take a moment to dive deep inside yourself.

With the mind of a beginner, examine how you feel. Why do you feel the way you do? Where are you overly invested? What might need to change about how you view those around you, how you view life, how you view yourself? What would you rather *not* to be true so that you can continue feeling unchallenged, so you don't have to change?

Use the book as an opportunity to move beyond your own limitations.

Your body and your life are reflective of and relative to the amount of stress, tension, and distortion you're holding inside. If you want to expand beyond your limitations, especially the limitations of your mind, you have to go into the body to create profound, instantaneous, and permanent change. If you don't go into the body, your inner philosopher remains stuck with believing it can think its way into freedom. It isn't possible. Drop the idea now. It's complete bulls--t.

I'm your tour guide into this new world, and I'm not here to be liked. What I care about is that you get the sobering truth that no one gave me. You may not agree with it, though you cannot question what's available here.

If you're scared, address it head-on. You may need additional support or education to help you move through your limitations and fears. Do the vulnerable thing and reach out. As you'll notice from my journey, reaching out for help was extremely uncomfortable, yet I did, and my whole life changed for the better.

You can look forward to being free and realizing other choices are available to you. You can become comfortable in body, increase your emotional and intellectual intelligence, eat and sleep and digest better. Every aspect of your life can become better with less effort because you'll get a deeper dynamic experience of your life.

If you don't want that, put the book down. Burn it. Go back to pretending you got it all together.

If you do want to be free, then you have one choice: you must take out the unresolved stress, tension, and distortion. Only then can you begin to access a fuller, greater expression of who you really are and leave the hell of struggle, strife, and suffering and upshift into ease and grace.

For the true seekers who resonate with freedom as part of their life's purpose, read this book a minimum of three times. Regardless of your level of intelligence, it'll take a minimum of three reads to fully integrate what's being offered.

With the greatest amount of humility, I wish you luck on your journey to discover freedom from the inside out.

INTRODUCTION

A PAINFUL JOURNEY

At twenty-two, I was a Navy SEAL in my prime. I was at a sleek 1.8 percent body fat and could run three miles in under fifteen minutes. I worked out all day long at a very high level. I could outperform professional athletes. Pound for pound, I was one of the strongest people on the planet. In terms of sheer fitness, I was the dictionary definition of peak condition. Yet after seven years of being a Navy SEAL and going through that intense training and performance, there was one problem: I was terribly unhealthy. You may wonder, how could a person who exercises rigorously be unhealthy? I didn't have the awareness yet to understand that the answer is in the question.

Health is something that begins internally and is then reflected on the outer body, whereas fitness is evident externally, but gives no indication as to what's going on under the hood. Fitness can be measured in cardiovascular numbers, examining how well the heart handles demands from the muscles' actions, as well as body-to-fat ratio. But these figures do not reflect the *health* of one's body. Health is not six-pack abs, it's far more.

In my experience, the people who are the most fit tend to be some of the unhealthiest people in the world. Fit bodies often mask hidden dangers. Fit people simultaneously have a lot of tension and stress in their systems. The health of their tissues, their range of motion, and their under-the-surface issues are far from optimal.

I often say that it would be easier for me to take a couch potato and develop a functional body than it would be to take someone who's been involved in athletics for a lifetime and try to build a functional body from there.

The so-called fit individuals I work with in my health practice tend to house the most stressors in their bodies. This surprises them, especially because they've spent a significant amount of time doing physical activities like heavy weight lifting and yoga. These are often very successful people who've incorporated stress into their lives and essentially play through it.

STRESS + TIME = *STRAUMA*

Piled-up stress causes severe and traumatic damage over time—what I call, "strauma," a combination of stress and trauma. If you add a tiny amount of stress every day, it adds up. After fifteen straight years, you'll eventually have a neglected body that reflects the entirety of all that harm.

In fact, most human beings on this planet walk around with bodies that are highly traumatized. This is why we can walk by each other and not even manage a smile when someone says hello. This is how we can yell with such hatred and bile at someone in the car next to us who also just wants to get home. We all become trapped in toxic bodies that are nothing more than dry powder kegs. We're like frogs slowly being boiled alive. We don't notice the heat at first, because it's not so bad that we jump out of the pot and it rises just steadily enough that we endure it until we no longer can.

I've had friends who are the picture of fitness bend over to tie a shoe only to wind up face-down in pain on the ground, having blown out their lower back. Next thing they know, they're in bed for three or four weeks, trying to figure what on Earth happened. Anyone involved in athletics learns early on an old adage: mind over matter. In other words, choose to override the pain that your body is feeling. Add to that the motto of the SEALs, "If you don't mind, it doesn't matter," and you end up ignoring every warning signal your body sends out. Eventually, the message will sink in, and when it does, it will be too late. Your body will have suffered tremendous damage by then.

When I was the poster boy for fitness, I had pain in every joint, in my feet, knee, shoulder, wrist, lower back, and neck. I needed a full-blown hip replacement at age thirty-three. I was reading lips because my hearing was shot, and my vision was rapidly going, as well. On top of that, I was getting up five to ten times a night to pee and was a zombie-like insomniac.

These are all symptoms anyone living a typical life in an industrialized country has experienced at one point or another. Mine were just exacerbated by the intensity of my youthful endeavors. I was running on adrenaline rather than the proper energy my body should have been creating from nutrients. I was taxing my adrenal glands, which wears out joints and exhausts the nervous system. Everything I had done in my life was now affecting my body.

IF IT'S IN YOUR BODY, IT'S IN YOUR LIFE

After the SEALs, I began training for the Olympics in track and field. Every two or three months, however, I would be beset by another nagging injury. In fact, I kept becoming more and more susceptible to injuries in large part because I had but one gear. I gave 100 percent to everything I did. If I had a "turbo" button that allowed me to do 110 percent, I was using it. While others around me paced themselves, chose their battles wisely or found other reasons to train at some level under their highest potential, I left it all on the field every time.

I used to admire the older runners, whose knees were extensively taped and who grimaced with every step. "That guy's hardcore," I would think. There is something written into our mythology as Americans which glorifies the stoic man who suffers in silence. We tell legends of such men.

Ours is a culture that honors only the winners, not the second-place finishers. You've probably heard: "Second place is first loser," or seen it on a T-shirt at the gym. In any endeavor, be it finance, sports, or the arts, we only devote our attention to the very best in the field. The others have failed, as far as our society is concerned. It's not surprising, then, that we fail to document the torment that people go through in their attempt to reach the top. Nor do we focus on the physical agony that takes a toll on the bodies of those who strive for success.

To do so, as a society, would be to bear some responsibility in the unnecessary maiming of our sons and daughters.

When you look at events like the Olympics, what you see is triumphant. In twenty years, there will be another batch of victorious athletes doing amazing things. But this generation of athletes, meanwhile, will be battling the most difficult physical challenges of their lives, not on a pommel horse or a diving platform, but getting out of bed or bending their knees. They are accumulating strauma that they will pay for later.

The strauma that occurs in life will eventually manifest in the body. If we keep stressing ourselves out, it will eventually turn into pain, fatigue, depression, or more.

I worked with an Olympic medalist in synchronized swimming who faces those challenges today. Nobody told her that a few years after her moment of glory, she would be dealing with an eating disorder that affects her before, during, and after every meal. But hey, when she competed, she looked terrific in a swimsuit and won a bronze medal. It must be worth it.

The attitude of our society is work hard, achieve greatness, don't worry about tomorrow. Give it 100 percent all day, every day. Go all out. There is no need for balance, because the medal, the recognition, the signing bonus, is worth the pain. Nobody is going to pay you a six-figure income to be a well-rounded human being who just does solid work every day. You have to be exceptional. There

is no reward for being a well-adjusted, emotionally intelligent, or spiritually developed person.

I can only imagine the amount of strauma the world's
all-time most successful Olympian, Michael Phelps, has
accumulated. He's matured a great deal now and is a
father, but there was a time when he was smoking marijuana, getting into trouble, in car accidents, and fights
with his girlfriend. He would train eight hours in the pool,
then brag about eating McDonald's three times a day. His
body might've burned calories like a furnace, but there's
a lot more to nutrition than just calorie count. He may
have been perfectly fit, but, most likely, he was also perfectly unhealthy.

Life is very much like a golf swing: if you have something
in your life that is causing a figurative hitch in your swing,
you might be able to tweak your mechanics and get the
ball on the fairway most of the time, but it isn't the optimal, long-term solution for healthy living. Eventually,
you'll rupture a lumbar disc or strain a ligament. Wouldn't
it be better in the long run to simply fix your life swing?

FROM SEALING TO HEALING

I've spent the last seventeen years getting healthy from
the inside out rather than the outside in. I was tired of the
pain and ready to discover a new way to live. For the first

seven years, I employed different healing methodologies to discover what worked and what did not. There were times where I spent upwards of six hours a day working on myself, doing things like acupuncture, stretching, fasting, massages, and colonics. I became an investigator into my own health. I gathered information and looked at the data. I analyzed, categorized, and synthesized everything I learned to find the connections that would eventually lead to my own healing.

During the seven years that I spent gauging my recovery, I was constantly monitoring my health. I developed a data-gathering process to measure my results. Furthermore, I wanted to know if those results were unique to me or if I could apply what I'd been learning to help others. It turns out that I could do exactly that.

The level of health I've achieved is now my default state of being. It's a state of freedom from emotional and physical pain. I call it "Free for Life," and anyone can attain it by following the co-creative healing system that I've devoted the latter half of my life developing: True Body Intelligence.

What I have discovered, developed, and refined is something that was not even possible a mere decade ago: rapid and permanent change. If you look closely at your life and you see something that is not working the way you want it to, I guarantee you there is a place where you have some level of stagnation in your body that reflects exactly what you are experiencing, because whatever is in your body, is in your life.

To make sure that the process does, in fact, work, I took the next seven years off completely: no acupuncture, no fasting, no exercise, no stretching, no running, no lifting, no massages. Contrary to common wisdom, my body kept getting better. I went from working about four to five hours a day to sixteen, stress-free. I could wake up after just four or five hours of sleep and be wide-eyed and ready to go. I truly was free for life.

Free for Life is an opportunity to get your life back together from the inside out. It is about attaining freedom. Freedom from stress; freedom from tension; freedom from trauma; freedom from distortion; freedom from delusions. This is a process of being present in your life, which leads ultimately to a deep sense of happiness that has its basis in *you*, rather than your external circumstances. It's about re-wiring your system from the inside out and from the ground up.

I work from the standpoint of and draw inspiration from the Bruce Lipton book, *The Biology of Belief*, in which he makes the compelling case that what you believe, you achieve. If you doubt that a healthy state of being is possible for you, that disbelief is the first toxic substance that you must rid yourself of. Most people don't even realize that what they believe is based on what their parents and grandparents experienced. It isn't even their own belief system, yet they keep believing it.

In fact, human beings will even ignore data that they have collected, to stay loyal and devoted to limiting belief systems. This denial of reality has an evolutionary benefit, or it would've been scrapped long ago. The reason it survives, and even thrives, is because a person receives a sense of gratification from remaining true to a belief or a belief system even in the face of information to the contrary. We please our parents, for instance, by following their values even if we understand that they are outdated or outright wrong.

There is no room for that kind of unreality in my program. For me, it's simple: I apply the scientific method to everything. If it's real, then it's real. Data doesn't lie. I'm a Navy SEAL. I do practical and simple. I find the root of the problem, and I sort it out. This is what I'm here to help you do. You are in control; I am simply here as your guide.

It is up to you to take the first step and take responsibility for your own health. If you don't recognize something as being broken, then there is no fixing it. It can be difficult for people to take ownership of their own road to recovery.

I needlessly entered a world of pain and suffering because I adopted belief systems that weren't true to who I was as a person. Instead, I learned to project an image that others wanted to perceive in me. I wasn't ready to recover, until the pain was too unbearable. As I see it, my job is to connect to you in the deepest way possible so that we can work together in a common pursuit so that you never reach a point of unbearable pain.

We will work in conjunction to achieve a desired goal. Co-creation involves two parties. In this way, you aren't merely unloading a pile of problems on someone only to go home depressed and start drinking. Neither are you obsequiously waiting for that other person to bring you gift-wrapped solutions to your problems. On the contrary, this method requires cooperative effort from both sides to connect and in that synergy, build a transformative solution to the problem. And it's a learning experience for both sides.

This, of course, is antithetical to the way the American educational system has taught us to learn. At its best, it uses a teacher-student model, which is fine for some purposes, such as learning math or history. At its ugliest, it is an institution designed to coerce children into obedience to authority. Either way, it produces a nation of guru-worshippers who are dependent on someone else to solve their problems.

Ultimately, my system is just that, a system. There's a structure that provides a way to proceed. It's a two-way process that relies on us working together in a co-creative manner. As such, it is something that allows people to direct their attention through, but it will not do anything unless you are willing to put in the work. Eventually, as you begin to achieve self-mastery, you must walk away from the system and listen to the dictates of the moment.

True Body Intelligence will give you the tools to become independent of the images you've been taught to project, and for which you've been "rewarded" with the opportunity to conform with the larger society. With that independence comes self-empowerment. Rather than give you fish, we show you how to fish.

This process involves shaking some well-entrenched habits along the way, and requires a re-education of the body, brain, and nervous system. It requires deconditioning the body from stress and from seeking approval from others rather than from within. It's easier said than done, of course. I've worked with some of the most successful people in the world, top artists, actors, athletes, writers, producers, directors, musicians. They are externally successful human beings who don't have a clue who they are. And they are miserable inside.

The greatest tragedy of our era is the loss of self. It's happening on a pandemic scale, but people don't even realize that it is happening, because it happens so slowly as they chip away a little bit of their real selves every day, buying into a false image of who they think others want them to be.

If this sounds like you, here's how this book can help: as you read, highlight everything that makes you feel uncomfortable with a bright yellow marker. It's the places where you feel uncomfortable which are going to produce the greatest amount of shift in your limiting belief systems.

In ten thousand years, human beings will have a far greater understanding of reality, including these bodies, and we will be able to target any pain and diagnose its cause immediately. But before that can happen, we have to rewire ourselves from the inside out. That's why I wrote this book.

Part I

THE JOURNEY
TO TRUE BODY
INTELLIGENCE

CHAPTER 1

A YOGA MAT AND A JUICER

If I had to pinpoint a day in which my journey to true body intelligence began, it would be a day in 1999 when I was in an incredible amount of pain all over my body, particularly in my joints. I called my Navy SEAL buddy, Jeff Higgs, and told him about it. He replied in his Staten Island accent, "Yo Chris, don't worry man. I'll be right over and I'm going to bring a yoga mat and a juicer."

I had no idea what he was talking about. I told him I didn't know what a yoga mat was but said I could go to the grocery store if he wanted some OJ or apple juice. He laughed hysterically and told me to sit tight.

He showed up about thirty minutes later with two yoga

mats, a big stainless-steel contraption, and a bag of produce: carrots, celery, parsley, beets, apples, lemons, and ginger.

"Your tissues are toxic," he told me. Again, I had no idea what the heck he was saying.

He was in the kitchen chopping things and tossing them in the big steel juicer. And while he chugged his juice in about three or four minutes, I was still struggling to get mine down some forty-five minutes later. That's when it dawned on me: the reason he wasn't having a hard time with these raw fruits and vegetables was because he was healthy. I understood in that moment that my tissues were, indeed, toxic. Naturally, anything that tasted healthy to me was like taking medicine. On the other hand, artificial foods had, over the years, begun to taste normal.

Jeff understood where I was at, physically. We had endured SEAL training together and faced similar challenges due to our body type—we were both very lean. Because of that and because we spent so much time training in freezing water, we were both extremely susceptible to hypothermia. Jeff was also the person responsible for getting me back into school after the SEALs, as I attended college on the G.I. Bill. We had been through a lot together, so there was already a strong level of rapport and trust established when I got on the phone with him that fateful day in 1999.

Now, here we were on the floor of my apartment. Jeff demonstrated yoga postures for me to try, and, while I still tried to drink this strange fruit and vegetable juice, I could barely wrap my head around the fact that he was a human pretzel with a natural ability to contort his body. There was a point in time when our bodies could do the exact same things, but here he was crossing his arms over each other, bending his elbows, and getting his palms to touch. I could barely bring an elbow near its opposite shoulder. He called it eagle arms. I called it an exercise in futility.

I remember looking at him in frustration, thinking, "What the hell, he must have just been born that way." When I told him that, he laughed, then rolled onto his back and began cracking up even more. When I asked what was so funny, he told me that he used to be just as tight and stiff me, and unable to get into a basic posture. Then he told me he had begun dating a yoga teacher and got into it, practicing two to three hours a day over the last couple of years.

I began wondering where on earth I was going to come up with two or three hours a day. I wasn't sure if I could even manage one hour a day of yoga. Even if I could find the time, it hurt like hell and I wasn't so sure if I wanted to continue. However, when I woke up the next morning, I felt a little bit of relief. And I realized that if I didn't do something different in my life, I was going to continue living in the pain that haunted me every minute of the day regardless of what I was doing.

At the end of our first session, Jeff suggested I find a Rolfer. Yoga, he said, wasn't going to be enough for my pain. Once again, I had no idea what he was saying. A Rolfer, he explained, would do deep-tissue massage on my body, and they weren't shy about it, either. It wasn't going to feel good, but it was going to help the pain.

With Rolfing, I learned that one must learn to literally get the mind to relax the body regardless of how uncomfortable it might be. I had never used my mind for anything regarding my body except to push it to its limits. Rolfing was a wake-up call for me. I had spent thirty years of my life accruing damage to my body, and now I had to deal with that damage.

That day with Jeff, I had to face the fact that I simply wasn't healthy. The truth is, it's more than that. I believed that because I was fit, I was healthy, and I had to address that as a limiting belief. Equating fitness to health is not true, and now I didn't know what healthy was, yet I knew *I* wasn't healthy. Now I wondered, what is health?

The pain I experienced daily was evidence of my unhealthiness, yet I chalked up the pain to the rough-and-tumble life of a high-performing athlete. I assumed that the pain and the injuries I was experiencing were merely the product of an overachieving body. It couldn't possibly have anything to do with my behavior or my current lifestyle or even the trauma I experienced as a child. Could it?

THE ORIGINS OF THE PAIN

Before I could get better, I had to understand where all my pain originated from, and I knew the tension and stress in my body were not merely the result of hard athletic training. Other guys in the SEALs team had similar pains, yet not everyone was going through the same experience. I wondered how that was possible, and I began to realize the tension and stress was coming from somewhere else. My pain extended back long before I joined an elite military unit. In fact, it goes back even further than you might presume. It goes back to before I'd ever stepped foot into this world. It goes back as far as my time in the womb.

In 1968, tensions were high, Malcolm X had just been assassinated, Martin Luther King, Jr. had just been assassinated, Robert Kennedy had just been assassinated. There were race riots and the world was in turmoil.

My mother lived in a small town in the coal regions of Pennsylvania. She was Caucasian. And she was pregnant. My father was of mixed race. This was a problem because my great grandmother was an icon in town and my great uncle was the chief of police. I was an unmentionable secret even before I took my first breath of air.

My mother gave birth to me in Philadelphia and hid me there to be raised by others while she went back home. I had been born severely bow-legged. All the muscles in my body were pulling on my bones with so much force that it bowed my poor legs. On my second day on this earth, a doctor broke both my legs mid-thigh and had them placed in casts.

It solved the problem in the short run, to some extent. But the fix was essentially cosmetic. If someone is severely bow-legged, it means that their lateral hamstrings and iliacus muscles must be extremely short. But rather than take the tension out of the muscles in the fascia, their solution was to snap the bones in the legs and make them appear straight.

My childhood was a dark environment, and where I lived was regularly chaotic. The people I stayed with did drugs, consumed alcohol, and constantly yelled and screamed at each other. Fire became my escape. At three and a half years old, I knew how to light matches, because everyone in my house smoked. I used to strike a match, bring it up to my face, and watch as the flame burned down. I liked looking at the match because I could meditate on the light. At the time, I didn't have enough cognition to understand that the flame would eventually burn my skin. When I felt the heat, I would let go, say "Ow," and the match would hit my orange polyester rug and burn a black hole in it.

One time my mother was out, and I had a babysitter, a woman named Mrs. Baskerfield. She caught me lighting matches and she was angry. She came down the hallway screaming, picked me up, slapped the match out of my hand, and ran down the stairs to the kitchen with me slung onto her left hip.

I could feel the amount of rage coming through her as we moved through the house. She was a punisher and she used to throw me around when I did something wrong. Often, I would end up hitting my head and sustained a lot of traumatic brain injuries, but this day was worse, and I could feel it.

When we got to the kitchen, she lit the gas stove and said, "I'll teach you to never use matches again." Then she put my right hand on the fire. I fought to get the burning hand back and finally got free, but then she took my left hand and placed it in the flame, this time with more strength. My skin melted. Finally, I reached over and bit her. She dropped me on the floor, and I ran away.

As I left the room, I could hear her come to her senses and mutter, "Oh, my God, what the hell have I done?" She was in a state of shock. She ran to help me, then rubbed Vick's VapoRub on my burns. The pain was excruciating. All I remember is passing out and leaving my body. I sustained fourth-degree burns on my hands and became nearly comatose for three to six months.

After that, I learned to disappear. I didn't want to be seen, because I feared I would do something wrong and be punished. I learned to be in a room without anyone knowing I was there. My whole life, if I was ever in someone else's house, I would walk through a room they were in, and they would turn around and be startled. "Where the hell did you come from?" they'd ask.

Even though I was there, you couldn't feel me. I learned to keep my energy tied into me. When I crawled, I crawled quietly. I never cried. I never said much. I could come into your house and scare the pants off of you. These were all sophisticated mechanistic controlling strategies that I learned to employ at the age of three and a half and continued throughout my childhood.

I believed that if I could disappear and project to others the image they wanted to see, they wouldn't mess with me. Instead of being a cute puppy in a room that wanted attention, I was more akin to the stuffed animal on the bed. You'd look at me and think, oh he's cute, but you wouldn't interact with me and I wouldn't interact with you.

I was so pulled into myself that whole parts of my personality didn't form to be in a way that was relatable to the outside world. I became over-adaptable to my environment. I didn't say "no, I won't do that" or "I don't like that" or "leave me alone"; I went along with everything.

In fact, there were a couple years in my childhood where I basically didn't say a word. I only did as I was told. During that time, there was a lot I wanted to say, but I held it in. Finally, when I did speak up, it came out with so much heat on it that it felt like I was crushing people. I was almost like a scorpion. I would stun people, because they would think, "Look, he's so nice, he's adapting." And then I would let them have it.

By the time I was seven, I was a full-blown stammerer. This was the year my mother passed away and they put me in the foster system. I couldn't speak, I couldn't get anything out, because I was struck from Post-Traumatic Stress Disorder (PTSD). You wouldn't know it if you saw me, but the second you asked me a question and I had to give you information, I stuttered.

This happened because I went from being able to disappear and only having to deal with people one on one to suddenly being in a boarding school. Now, I was surrounded by fifteen other kids plus the house parents and their two kids in a student home.

THE MILTON HERSHEY SCHOOL

When my mother passed away, I ended up at an amazing institution called the Milton Hershey School. It was founded and run by Milton Snavely Hershey and his wife, Catherine, in 1909 and was designed for so-called "unfortunates," children who had lost their fathers in war. Here, it was impossible to disappear.

I was fortunate that two of my house parents looked out for me. They were a married couple named Bub and Cleta Aikens. On the first day at the house, Cleta realized I stammered and invited all the boys in to see. She said, "Christopher, can you say something?"

I responded, "Ye-, ye-, ye, ye-, yes, mm-, mm-, Mrs. Aikens."

She told the boys, "This boy's a stammerer, and if I ever hear any one of you make fun of him, you will be on the gravy train."

Everyone knew what the gravy train was and no one

wanted to be on it. If you were on the gravy train, you were doing the dishes of twenty people, cleaning the floors, the sinks, and the counters while all the other boys were out playing. It was a big job and you would end up cleaning from 5:30 to 8:30 at night. You'd have one hour to do your homework and then it was bedtime. None of the boys wanted to be on the gravy train, so no one ever teased me.

The school sent me to a speech therapist named Mister Mullard who helped me learn to breathe, and because no one made fun of me, the stutter eventually started to go away. Later, I realized that the emotional body controls the breath and my emotional body was completely underdeveloped. In the moment, however, I learned that if I wanted to speak, I had to breathe. If I wasn't breathing, I wasn't getting enough air, and it was impossible for me to relax and allow words to move through me. Breathing and subsequently speaking allowed me to begin to self-express authentically. However, that didn't mean things were perfect.

When you're raised in an institution like I was at Milton Hershey School, everything is based on your efforts, your conduct, and your behavior. It's all rules and regulations, and your whole existence is based on the merit system. If your room was clean, you got a merit. If you did a chore well, you got a merit. If you were dressed appropriately, you got a merit. If you had a good attitude, which means you didn't talk back or question anything, you got a merit. If you had earned a certain number of merits at the end of the week, certain extracurricular freedoms and privileges and activities would be available.

By that same token, if your performance was less than satisfactory, you would be issued a demerit. And as you can surmise, demerits were associated with punishments. The entire system is based on creating and encouraging obedience to authority through the experience of cause and effect. *I do this, I get that; I don't do this, I don't get that.*

The long-term result of the merit system and, for that matter, institutionalization, however, is that I was never able to get in touch with my own notions of right and wrong behaviors. When you have parents who are raising you and you share their biology, if you push back or misbehave, you might get into trouble but chances are, they're not going to send you away. That is the underlying threat that an institutionalized child always faces.

For the most part, I was a good kid, which is to say I sought to earn merits, garner approval, and stay out of trouble. I lived on the dairy farm portion of the school. That meant getting up a little before 5:30 each morning and preparing for barn, as we called it, which entailed milking the cows, shoveling manure, and other farm tasks. We were each required to spend two weeks doing a job on the dairy farm, then two weeks back at the house. Two weeks later, it would be back to the dairy farm to perform a different task.

They always kept circulating us through all the different types of chores. At first, I hated barn because I'm very sensitive in terms of my sense of smell and hearing. I was also the kid that would never get in the sandbox because I didn't like the feel of the grains of sand touching my skin, and barns were dirty. But there was no way out of the chores; it was part of the system that I had to learn to deal with. This was when I learned to put my own needs aside. By the time I was a junior, barn was just another part of life.

My experiences at the Milton Hershey School prepared me for joining the SEALS. In addition to the merit system and ignoring the discomfort of the dairy farm, the students' homes consisted of groups of sixteen students. Among them, four were officers. Guess how many people constitute a SEAL team? Yep, sixteen. And four of them are officers.

I understood the dynamics of that structure because I had been living it as long as I could recall. That arrangement, which was foreign to most people, was what I called home. Despite the shortcomings of the institutionalization, the

Milton Hershey School was a good place to grow up for a kid without a lot of options.

I didn't have a lot of choice in my upbringing. I had an elderly grandmother back home who didn't have the energy to properly raise me, and there was nowhere else to go. I had to make school work. That meant that I had to sacrifice some of my own desires to maintain good standing.

I was rather invulnerable because I didn't have anybody there that I cared for, and the way that the school was set up, house parents had to give all the children the same level of attention; they couldn't show favoritism. Everyone got the same cake on their birthday: the same flavor, the same shape, the same color. Everyone got the same birthday card. Everything was always the same.

In the meantime, the only interaction we had was with each other. In that way, it was a brutal place. We all tended to come from similarly bad circumstances. We'd all lost a parent or both parents, maybe the family was in dire straits financially. Whatever the case, kids can be cruel to each other, especially when they know the pain points of their peers.

It was very difficult to find someone at the school that would put loving attention into you. The kids who flourished were the ones who knew how to read the social cues. I wasn't among them. I had to soothe myself at night. There were a lot of tears when the lights went out. I had to take care of myself emotionally. Once you learn to soothe yourself, eventually, you don't need anyone to soothe you.

I had become a hardened human being. By lighting my hands on fire at a young age, Mrs. Baskerfield had done more damage than what was visible on my skin. Of course, I didn't know this at the time, but as I began my journey to health, I would soon understand its full impact.

TRIAL BY FIRE AND WATER

Fire was the first element I was introduced to on the planet, and it went straight into my skin and my body. In Chinese medicine, the two meridians that are impacted the most on both hands are the lung and large intestine. The large intestine is the channel for ambition. The lung is the channel for perfection, completion, power, boundaries, and truth. They both represent the element of metal.

Mrs. Baskerfield had put fire in my metal channels. In a way, she made me into a sword—a power for ambition and perfection.

I was no longer a malleable young child made of soft

metal that could still be impacted by his environment; I was a knight in armor, impenetrable. The hardships of life didn't affect me, because my metal was forged by the flame on the stove.

I couldn't feel the full effect of my environment and life on my body. Throughout childhood, I remained disconnected. Fortunately for me, I had a high IQ, so I could learn quickly, but most of the time I was off in another place, no matter where I was. When I was in SEAL training, I was numb to life. I couldn't feel the energetic, emotional, and mental impact that life had on me, and I became alone. In a certain way, SEAL training was a joke. It was hard in terms of the effort, because you must put out a lot of energy, but if I was struggling and I was bothered by anything that was going on, I couldn't feel it anywhere because I didn't know me. That "me" was under the armor, and my armor was so strong that people couldn't reach me.

I couldn't take feedback from anyone. The only person who could speak to me about me was me. I was shielded by a thick metal wall and anything said to me about me bounced right off. I had no issue sharing wisdom or advice, but I could never take it in.

As I grew older, this impacted my relationships, especially the personal and romantic ones. In those relationships people want communication and vulnerability, but I could never offer this. Instead of being vulnerable, I became a manager of everyone around me.

I needed to be in control of my environment. I had learned that if I could manage the amount and kind of information I gave to others, then I could avoid punishment, rejection, humiliation, and violence. I would only give the information partners wanted to hear, so they could never call me out on anything. Technically, everything was fine, but it was a terrible place to be.

I was incredibly ambitious, but to be successful you must be vulnerable. You have to communicate clearly your wants, desires, and needs. Because I could never be vulnerable, I lacked the ability to communicate my needs.

I became stoic because my needs were never met.

I was anesthetized and I had no idea growing up how deeply that one incident at the age of three and a half had affected my entire being. Too much fire in my metal hardened my armor. It turned it into Excalibur. Even though I might experience pain—physically, mentally, emotionally, psychologically, energetically—I didn't feel the impact at the time, and it would only get worse.

Fire ignited in my body at the age of three and a half, but

its opposite, water, had no place to go. That flame heated up all the metal within, but my water became stagnant and all that cold got trapped inside that metal. I was constantly cooling down on the inside. It wasn't until I was twenty-two and began training for the SEALS where I would feel the full effects of this.

The athletic training was easy, but the part that tested me the most in SEAL training was what they called surf torture. During this water training we'd wear nothing but cotton clothes and sit in the ocean water which was at 50-53 degrees, at 4:00 in the morning. The wind would whip around us and cool us even further, and then we'd have to do pull-ups and other training while soaking wet.

My body, a body that was already holding in the cold within its tough metal exterior, froze.

On my first attempt through hell week, I was hospitalized for full-blown hypothermia. We were training at the marine base in Oceanside, California, in December. On a Wednesday, we had finished our water torture and were sitting around a fire. Guys were telling jokes left and right and having a good time. I remember thinking that even though we had spent the day in the cold-water training, I was incredibly warm. After a few hours, we got up to leave and one of the instructors looked over at this maze of oars and said, "If anyone knocks one of those over, you guys are going right back down to the ocean and we're going to surf torture you all night long."

Every other guy got up and walked through the oars without a problem. I was the last to go and knocked down every single oar. Then I remembered, as a kid, I loved watching the National Geographic channel and one of the episodes that stuck in my head was one about Eskimos. They talked about hypothermia and described how Eskimos know that if they get too far away from home and they're not reading the signs correctly and a storm comes in, the Eskimo will die of hypothermia. One of the last things they feel before they die is extremely warm.

I had spent the day in cold water, and a lifetime of trapping the cold in my metal exterior, yet here I was stumbling to bed feeling extremely warm.

One of my buddies, said, "man, how are you doing?" I said, "Dude, I'm so warm. I'm so warm." And he was like, "I'm freezing, how the hell can you be warm?"

And then it hit me. I remembered that TV show. I said, "Uh-oh, that thing's happening." The instructor staff had to pull down my pants and give me a thermometer in my rectum because they needed to measure my core temperature.

It was 87.4 degrees. My heart went into ventricular fibrillation, which is basically a heart attack. They rushed me to the hospital and slowly introduced me into a hot tub to bring me back to a normal 98.6 degrees.

Looking back, I now know that excessive heat had hardened my body and trapped in the excessive cold. I lived on the extreme ends of the spectrum. I could experience anything within that range and it didn't affect me. Other people are horrified by certain things because they have a limited range of what they can experience. For me, my limits were so broad and deep that I had room and space for anything to happen around me, and I was okay with it. I almost died, yet I said I was fine.

LOSING BALANCE

At twenty-nine, I lost 50 percent of my hearing because my kidneys got too cold, and my heart too hot.

I was out of balance.

In Chinese medicine, the kidneys are the center for water and cold. The heart's the center for fire and heat. The kidneys' job is to cool down the heart, but my heart was too hot and my kidneys were too cold. The extreme heat and extreme cold were trapped within my body and they didn't cancel each other out, instead they continued to intensify.

As I got hotter, my kidneys had to provide more cold. My kidneys, now overtaxed, began to run out of energy, so they started stealing energy from all the other organs to keep that furnace in my chest cooled down.

By the time I was thirty-one, I had ankle, knee, low back, shoulder, and neck pain, and it was continuous. My joints were seizing up, but I was still carrying on like everything was fine.

I didn't have the ability to inform anyone that I was suffering underneath. Reaching out to Jeff Higgs that day was a huge step. To admit out loud that I was in pain was incredibly difficult, but it was a great first step.

I had been holding so much behind that metal shield, because I was invulnerable, that it was causing intense physical pain.

In some way, having those two extremes made me unpredictable because I could swing into whatever environment I was in. I could swing into whatever needed to be done, and at the highest level of doing it. If something needed to be done well, I did it really, really well. It also meant that when you came into my environment and into my home, I had to control the environment. The shoes had to be here, the coats had to be there, the dishes had to look like this, the pillows had to be in the right place on the couch. If they were any different, then things would get crazy. Everything needed to be in the perfect, logical space for me to feel comfortable and safe. *OCD*

My ambition at that time was to achieve my goals. Rather than figure out who I wanted to be, I was focused on what I wanted to do.

I was not concerned about the journey or the experience, I was only focused on the goal.

If you're only focused on the end point, you're not focused on the impact you have on your environment and the people around you. I was forcing everyone to over-adapt into what I did, because I had the cold inside.

I had fixed ways of thinking, being, communicating, relating, and emoting, and things got too compartmentalized.

I'd come up with these ideas of what that meant. "What does it mean if I'm a doctor? What does it mean if I'm a Navy SEAL? What does it mean if I go to the Olympics?" For me, I equated a bronze or silver or a gold medal as a display of winning at life. That I somehow had achieved value and importance.

But the thing is, I might have been winning at achieving, but I was losing at being.

When I first attempted yoga with my friend Jeff Higgs, I couldn't get into any of the positions, because I was hardened like steel. He was a soft, malleable structure, and I looked like a DeLorean. I was a cool car that looked good, but I was just stainless steel.

I couldn't get into any of the positions with Jeff, but I was always more fit than him because underneath I had so much fire. I could outrun him, out-swim him, and out-do him. I could push past discomfort because I didn't feel it. I had no idea I was harming my body.

But I was fit as hell.

I could keep pushing into the pain and the discomfort, but I had lost my flexibility and range of motion. Within that limited amount of flexibility and range of motion, I was an enraged wood-burning furnace, and I was ambitious. I was determined to get to the other side. To accomplish grapevine arms and all the other poses Jeff demonstrated with ease.

Looking back, I realize I still had a lot to learn. I may have been working towards softening my body, but the rest of me was still frozen and unmovable.

I had gotten the goal, but I hadn't figured out, at all, what I wanted to experience along the journey. I was an empty shell. A beautiful bronze state on the outside, hollow on the inside. I was the DeLorean that rides up to the restaurant and turns eyes, but sputters to a stop five minutes after it pulls out of valet.

The trial by fire and water shut my system down. It caused me to lose my vision, my hearing, my mobility, and my body's ability to feel comfortable and repair, in a twenty-four-hour period.

Here I was: a super-fit guy on the outside, but incredibly frail on the inside.

I couldn't allow anyone to attach to my pain, and so it was stuck because I wasn't vulnerable enough to receive help. I could only live in silence with my pain.

There's a saying in SEAL training: "If you don't mind, it doesn't matter." Basically, it meant that if you don't mind the sensation and feeling of pain and discomfort, then keep moving on as if nothing is wrong with what you're experiencing.

It gave me permission to hurt myself more. I learned to suck it up and persevere, but you can only do that for so long before you crack.

The wounds caused by the fire and the water were bound

to be felt, and that's what would ultimately happen. A pendulum can only swing so far in one direction before it comes back the other way.

When you live your life in avoidance, whether it be avoidance of humiliation, rejection, punishment, or anything else, you slowly lose your authentic identity and develop a false sense of self. Your personal identity disappears. Admitting the pain to Jeff was the first step in coming back to myself. Starting yoga was just the beginning. I had no idea how long the journey would be or that the pain would get worse before it got better.

CHAPTER 2

WEEKEND AT ROBERTO'S

Everything came to a head when I was in a car accident at the age of thirty-two. I had driven into an intersection on a green light when a car came barreling down a hill at high speed. The brakes went out as it neared the light and the car struck the passenger side of my car and spun it around, careening me into a light post. The car was damaged, and so was my body.

Imagine if you took a car and filled it with thick glass, and suddenly it was in an accident. The whole thing would shatter. This was my hardened body. Upon impact, I shattered. Everything that was already steeled inside me burst into the deepest parts of my being.

I had been in pain prior to the accident, but that crash put me over the edge. Before, I felt my pain most intensely on the outside part of my hip and had been doing yoga to treat it. However, after the crash, my pain shifted deep inside and I felt that I would never get away from it. I had reached a place of unbearable pain.

After the accident, I was in need of pain relief, and I knew that I needed more than yoga. I began to combine a variety of treatments.

I started with Rolfing. Jeff had told me to research Rolfing, but it took me seven to eight months to find the right person.

I had run into a buddy from boarding school in San Diego and he invited me to a party in Laguna Niguel the next day. The party was not like the parties I was used to, where people were drinking, tossing a Frisbee, hanging out, discussing sports. Here, everyone was talking about love and light, and I started to wonder what I had stepped into. But I was having a good time, so I embraced the experience.

For months prior to this party, I had interviewed Rolfers, but no one seemed right and I wasn't ready to shell out a significant amount of money until I knew I had the right person. Then I met Steven Bulger.

He was at the party and he explained that his technique was not the original technique created by Ida Rolf. Instead he practiced Hellerwork, which was founded by a guy named James Heller who had created his own school after studying with Ida Rolf. He explained the differences, and they made sense to me.

Steven was a spiritual guy. He wasn't the guy at the party that was drinking; he was communicating and connecting with everyone and laughing, and he made me feel comfortable.

The next week I went to my first session with Steven, and I filled out the paperwork that chronicles your pain and other disease history. Then he sat me down in a little chair and he said, "Who are you?" I thought it was a weird question, but I answered, "I'm an athlete."

He said, "You're an athlete?"

I said, "Yeah. I'm an athlete."

"Are you sure about that?"

And I said, "Yeah. I'm an athlete."

He said, "Well, here at the top of your sheet it says you're Christopher Lee Maher. You might want to think about that for a second." And then he left the room.

I thought, "This mofo. Who the hell does he think he is? What is this psycho-babble nonsense? I didn't come down here for this. I came down here to get rid of this pain in my body so I can get back to training."

It pissed me off. I was not happy that he went there, and a part of me wanted to get out of the office and leave, but there was another part of me that knew this guy was the right guy and I knew it was the right situation. However, at the same time, I didn't want someone to look at my inner deficiency. I wanted to keep avoiding that part of me. I wanted to avoid looking at what he was saying because I wanted to keep up with my own mindset.

At that time, I identified doing with success. What this guy was talking about was "being."

Because I'd become hyper-independent, I took a false pride in understanding who I was and what I was about, without letting anyone come in and question that. Steven was questioning my false identification, which was my status as an athlete.

There was a part of me that didn't want to change, that wanted to say, "Hey, get out of my face." And then there was a part of me that wanted to change. Fortunately for me, the part of me that did want to change was a little bit stronger than the part that wanted to avoid feeling humiliated.

He eventually came back in the room and we did the session, and it was good. When I got in my car, I was driving home, and of course the only thing that was on my mind was what he questioned. *Who are you?* I contemplated that question again and again and concluded that my over-identification with being an athlete is what drove me into the ground.

When I was younger, I got a lot of kudos for doing well in sports. I got to date the prettiest girls in high school. I got to go to college and have a good time being an athlete. Being an athlete was a reward, and I was always looking for that reward, but it was a false reward.

On that ride home I started looking over my history, and by the time I got home I knew Steven was right. I had identified with being an athlete. I called myself an athlete rather than Christopher.

It was then that I started to investigate into myself, why? And that brought up a whole slew of false assumptions that I had made, in terms of what was valuable about living, and the journey. He'd also taken an intense amount of stress out of my body, so now I had this spaciousness in myself to look at why my body was so tense. It was like a light had started to turn on and I never turned it off after that.

Steven and I went through our ten-session series, and by the end of that ten-session series, there were some differences and changes in terms of the stiffness within my joints and my range of motion.

The real value in our sessions was his questioning. *Who are you?* If you don't know who you are, you don't know why you're doing what it is you're doing. If you don't know why you're doing what you're doing, you can't question your motivations.

It's difficult to question "doing," because doing is so celebrated. Like, "Oh, he's an MD," or "He's in a successful position." But if you look at a lot of those people that have high levels of success, and you go behind closed doors with them, they're miserable human beings. I'm not saying they all are, but I'm saying there's plenty of them that are. At the end of the day, doing doesn't create any internal satisfaction and can never be a substitute for being. Being is the key to attaining inner freedom and outer peace.

After the car accident, I continued my sessions with

Steven. My insurance was willing to pay for some of my treatments and I didn't believe standard physical therapy would help me. So, I continued receiving Hellerwork, got acupuncture and deep-tissue massages, did yoga, and foam-rolled my body. After all this work, I started to feel more present.

I could see the levels of discomfort and pain in my joints was diminishing a bit, so I thought at the time that I was creating change. I also added a type of work called the Egoscue Method.

EGOSCUE METHOD

With the Egoscue Method, they give you what they call a menu. You come in, they take a picture of you, and they show you all the twists and turns in your body that are off, and then you get a menu. The menu consists of very specific groups of isolated exercises, and you get up and do this program for thirty minutes every single morning. I got up every morning, did my exercises, and felt great. But after a few months I thought, "Man I feel pretty good," so I took a day and a half off, and within a day and a half, the pain that I had before came back at the same level.

Then I thought, "Really? Are you kidding me? You mean I have to get up and do this the rest of my life?"

At that point I realized I wasn't creating real, permanent change; I was simply using band-aids to deal with the pain. The program certainly worked. If you didn't want to feel the pain that day, you just got up and did your menu. But the second you stopped your program, then the discomfort started creeping back in because the exercises could only address what you had on a surface level.

When I looked through the man who created Egoscue's book with a friend of mine, he helped me realize that the program was really for people who were sixty years old and above who'd never really exercised. Doing this thirty minutes every day would change **their** whole life. But for me, someone who had driven tension down into the deepest parts of my body, I needed something more. There was a point in my life when I didn't feel uncomfortable, and then suddenly all I felt was discomfort. I wondered, "How do I get back to that comfortable body I had before this discomfort and stiffness showed up?"

After my experience with the Egoscue Method, I started to realize the impermanence in the holistic community. I saw it with the Hellerwork. I saw it with the massages. I saw it with the acupuncture. I saw it with the yoga. I was doing all these things simultaneously, but they were basically band-aids.

I was incredibly frustrated. I was working my tail off and

every penny that I was earning I was spending on holistic care.

They all said the same thing, "Oh, listen, this is what this is going to do for you," and in the end if they told me that they were taking me a mile, the truth is they only took me a foot. Now I was happy for the foot, because the foot was a foot further down the road than I was before. Yet, I knew in my heart of hearts that there had to be something that created instantaneous permanent change. I used to say to myself, "God, you must've created one monkey on this planet that knows more than all these people added up together."

Don't get me wrong, these systems are great for a lot of people, but I knew I was different. I knew I had extenuating circumstances. Ninety-nine point nine percent of the planet has never been through something like SEAL training. They've never been through the levels of physical trauma that I experienced by the age of three and a half. The holistic systems out there are okay for most people because their problem is on the surface, but mine was deep. It was right down where all that tissue connects to the bone. Theirs was in that soft muscle at the very surface. I had to come to grips with that and I knew there had to be something better. Every night, I called out for something to be sent to me.

FINDING THE ANSWER

About a year after my accident, my friend Mark and I went to visit another friend from boarding school named Justin, in Sedona, Arizona, where he lived. Mark knew about all my pain and the lengths I was going to heal myself.

Now, I didn't know much about Sedona before I went but Justin was a tour guide there, so he took us out to a secluded place where we could camp under the stars. Sedona is known as a spiritual place, but all I knew was that there was more magnetism in the Earth in that location and when planes flew overhead it messed with their compass. We get out there and suddenly under the moonlight, I started to have all these amazing realizations about life.

I was sitting around the fire, looking up at the sky, and started contemplating the celestial bodies. I thought, what's going on up there, and what's going on down here? They all have a relationship to each other based on size, density, and speed. Whatever's going on up there, must be going on down here. We are the stars. I put that to the back of my mind and a few days later, Mark and I headed back to San Diego.

Weeks later, Mark sent me an email. It said, "I just saw this guy on Good Morning America. He's got five stretches that will change your life."

At the time, I thought, "Mark, go screw yourself. Go find this guy and go stretch your brains out silly." I got this together. I'm doing the Egoscue Method, I'm doing Hellerwork, I'm doing yoga, I'm doing acupuncture, I'm doing deep-tissue massages, I got it. I thought, "Who is this guy? He comes to my house, I take him around everywhere for two weeks, showing him all over San Diego and Arizona—he's got a free vacation on me and what's he doing for me? He's sending me some dude that needs to change my life? No, Mark, you go change your life."

Initially, this offended me. Who does Mark think he is? I don't need anyone to help me. I can help myself. What I realized later was that I had created a life where I relied on hyper-independence. Mark offering help went against my own narrative. I didn't take kindly to people questioning my identifications.

Two weeks later, this sweet spiritual woman I knew who was an aesthetician called me and said, "Christopher, listen. I just saw this guy on Good Morning America."

I said, "Let me guess, he's got five stretches that will change my life?"

And she's like, "Did you see it?"

And I said, "No, I didn't see it but I'm starting to get the message. Yes, I'm starting to get the message."

The thing about me is I always waited for things to happen in threes. This was happening in twos, and then I heard the little voice in the back of my head that said, "Listen, Christopher. I need you to abandon this philosophy just one time, okay?" I was like, "Okay." So I got on the internet, and I started researching and reading everything I could about this guy. On his website, he had a lot of basic information, but the thing that stood out the most was that he had worked with Dara Torres.

He had just brought her back from the Olympics where she had won five medals at thirty-six years old. The thought in my head was, "Thirty-six-year-old women didn't typically win gold medals at the Olympics, let alone five. They were lucky if they came in tenth place. They didn't go and win two or three golds and a couple silvers." That caught my eye, and I said, "Oh, my God. He did that for this woman? Imagine what he could do for me."

As I read more into his website and learned about his methods, I remembered that when I was about seventeen, I'd had a vision of training with someone up in the mountains who knew what no one else knew, and that he would help me become the best version of myself. I had forgotten about that vision until this moment when

I began looking at his website and saw that he lived in the mountains.

On his site, he explained that a muscle's ability to shorten is directly proportional to its ability to lengthen. I realized that what he was essentially saying was that I was inflexible. That came as a shock to me. I didn't consider that my problem. I had injuries, not flexibility issues. In my head, I was flexible. I was incredibly fit. It didn't even dawn on me that lack of flexibility could be the cause of my problems until that moment.

So, I got down on the floor and attempted the five positions that were supposed to change my life. I couldn't get into a single one. I wasn't even close, and it wasn't for a lack of effort. I literally spent hours attempting to contort my body into these positions to no avail. It was very sobering. It was also a very freeing moment because I realized that it meant that there was hope that if I could get there, I might find relief. In spite of all the things I'd been learning, my first thought was the goal. I understood that this man might have the information and tools I could use to reach my goal of making it to the Olympic trials, with a shot at making the team. I had to work with him.

HUNTING HIM DOWN

Roberto was impossible to reach. I tried like hell to track

him down. I sent him emails, I made phone calls, I got in touch with his trainer. This went on for six whole months.

About the same time, I was thinking to myself, "Who was the idiot who invented the five-day work week?" I decided I was done with it. I shifted Friday out of my work schedule.

The first Friday I had off, I slept in and when I woke up, I looked down and saw my phone. All of a sudden, I thought, "I need to pray." Then I closed my eyes and put my hands together and prayed, "Dear God, give me some help. What more can I do? I emailed this guy. I called this guy. He doesn't pick up. This is nonsense. Can't you see I'm putting in honest effort here? Throw me a bone already."

Then I heard this little voice say, "Well, get up and call him now." I picked up the phone and dialed the center and Roberto himself answered. I said, "Listen. My name's Christopher Lee Maher. I've emailed you, I called you, you had a course, I had the resources, I wanted to sign up for the course, nobody got back to me. What kind of business do you run? You got tools out there, you could be helping me, and I'm sitting here suffering?"

He was taken off guard and said, "Whoa, hold on. Listen, I'm not helping anyone right now. I'm living in San Jose, and I'm working on my stretching method. I'm writing my book. And I'm growing my organic garden."

I thought to myself, "This guy's up in the mountains of San Jose and he's trying to grow a jungle in his back yard? And what the heck is organic? This can't be real," but I kept pushing into him.

Every time he came up with a "No," I had a new reason why the answer should be "Yes." After a while, and, I'm sure, much frustration on his part, he finally gave in: "Listen, I'll tell you what. I'm going to help you. I want you to call me back in three days."

I said, "Three days? For real? Based on my ability to get a hold of you now, three days might mean three years to you. What I'm going to ask you is, are we talking seventy-two human hours?" And he started laughing.

I told him, "Here's what I'm going to do. I'm going to sit in this apartment for three days. I'm not leaving. Okay? I'm not leaving until you call me."

He said, "Okay," and asked for my address.

Two days later, a book on traditional Chinese medicine arrived at my door. When I opened the package, I was so happy because I finally felt like there as an amazing human being who understood me. Anyone who was willing to help me out like this man was going to be my friend for life. In the book he wrote: "You know, the thing I didn't tell you when we were on the phone is, when I first heard your voice, I knew one day you would be famous."

At first I thought he was trying to feed into my ego, but I cast that aside and read the rest of the letter, and it was really honest. I had no idea that the thing that I would eventually become known for is working with people through the mindset of Chinese medicine and helping them get back into alignment, but this was the first step.

Roberto had included in the book a stretching position he'd drawn for me to try. He wanted me to test out the method before I went any further. I started experiment-ing right away. I got in this position and I started to work it, but I didn't know what the hell I was doing. All I could tell you was there was more pain in my thighs than I had ever experienced in my entire life, and then he wanted me to write him an exposé on what my experience was.

On the third day, he called and said, "Hey, my partner's out of town the first three weeks of June. You can pick one of those days between these three weekends." I picked June 7th, two days after my birthday. I got on a plane, went up there, met him at the airport, and he greeted me with a lot of love and kindness.

We went to his house and got started the next morning. That first day we did two four-hour sessions. He pushed and pulled on my body and used all these different techniques. When I woke the next morning, all the pain I had was gone except in the center of the hip. I'd had ganglion cysts on both of my wrists that had disappeared. The pain in my joints was gone.

I'd spent all the money I had up until this point trying to get this sort of relief and he provided it in one day. But let me be honest, the work was not easy. SEAL training was a cinch compared to this. Guys in the SEAL teams would never want to hear that, but it's the truth. SEAL training was easy. Any clown can put tension in their body. But taking the tension out? That's a completely different story and a whole new model for success that shifts you from doing into being, by dissolving lifetimes of accumulated tension, stress, and trauma.

When you're removing the tension, you have to feel all the emotions, feelings, upsets, and fears that you buried with that tension. You must walk back through every single door you came in. Imagine you have a piece of wood with pegs in it. In the center is the self and there's another path of the "not self." But you, as a human, keep jumping from peg to peg on a path further and further away from your authentic self. To get back to where you started at self, you have to retrace your steps and confront the false projections and assumptions you made up as you moved on in your personal journey.

You can't skip over a step. You literally must go back through the pegs, one at a time. For me, the tension and the pegs that I had to retrace were through my kidneys.

In our sessions, he would strip this intense amount of tension out of a part of my body and I would literally end up laughing like a hyena for twenty minutes, rolling around on the ground. The kidneys are the center for fear and nervousness, so all that nervousness and all that fear that I had buried into my body was now coming out, and it was coming out as laughter.

What I later learned was that the kidneys are the center for humor or seriousness. When I came in the door the first time, Roberto said, "Well, you know, you're a quite serious person."

I responded, "Yeah this is how it is. This is my philosophy. This is how life works." But that was another false assumption. What I discovered was that for me to be more humorous, the seriousness had to leave.

If you're dead-dog serious, you have a lot of tension and stress in the kidneys. The kidneys control the joints and the hearing. I had a lot of sedimentation, and my joints and hearing were suffering because of it.

So, there I was laughing, taking a big chunk of tension out of my body and at the end of the first day, he pulled me aside and said, "Listen, I got an idea. Would you be willing to stay four days?"

"Look man, I'd love to stay here and do more work, but I don't have any more money," I said.

"You don't need to pay me any more money," he said.

"Well, why do you want me to stay longer?" I asked.

"Look, I've been doing this for twenty-five years and I've never, ever seen anybody change this fast. And I need to know how you're doing it, so all the other people that I help can get to where you are as quickly as you're getting there," he said.

"Okay, if it helps other people, I'm down."

For the next four days, he worked on me three to four hours every morning and every evening. Every time he took out another layer of loaded tension, I laughed even more. Sometimes for as long as twenty minutes at a time.

If someone was recording me, they would have thought I needed to be put in an institution. But it was the best feeling. The whole time I was there, he was educating me more. He took me to the grocery store and showed me organic and bio-dynamic foods and taught me their benefits. Not only was the tension leaving my body, but I was also getting an education on how to continue caring for it. It was the best thousand dollars I ever spent.

AFTER THE MOUNTAINS

The amount of tension that left my body in those sessions with Roberto was incredible, but what happened after I left is even more incredible. While I was at Roberto's place in the mountains, I knew change was occurring, but because I was in a controlled environment I wasn't out relating with others, so I had no clue how much my personality and core vibration was changing as well. At that time, I had no idea that your personality changed when you took out tension. I had no idea that it was fear, trauma, and stress that put my tension in there. After the fourth day was over, I went to the airport and said my goodbyes. I was incredibly grateful. This man spent six to eight hours a day removing tension from my body. If I hadn't met him and removed that stress, tension, and distortion, my full life expression would be severely diminished. It isn't what you do know that hurts you, it's what you don't know.

By the time I got to the airport, enough of the tension I'd accumulated in my body from SEAL training and my childhood was gone that I no longer had pain in every joint, except for the little bit of pain that was still in the center of my hip, but that wasn't even the biggest change. When I walked through the airport, I had a completely different experience of reality than before I met Roberto. It used to be that when I walked through the airport people would always step out of my way incredibly fast. It didn't matter who was walking toward me. It could be an NFL linebacker and they would still step to the side when I walked toward them. No one ever bumped into me. I always thought it was weird, but I never thought much more than that.

However, after four days with Roberto, as I walked through the airport, people were bumping into me left and right. I took note that this was even weirder than before and when I got on the plane, I ended up in the four seats that faced each other. This was back when Southwest Airlines had the first two front rows facing backward and the next two facing forward, so it was like you were in a train cabin and you were facing your neighbors. Normally, when I got on a plane people would immediately move their arm off the armrest and keep to themselves, but this time people started talking to me. They were interested in what I did and who I was. We conversed the entire flight home and it was a wonderful new experience.

When I got in the taxi to head home in San Diego, I felt a new spaciousness inside of me to experience everything that I already knew in a completely different way. I had lived in the city for ten years and knew the lay of the land, but now I was in love with every tree and hillside we drove by. I had so much gratitude for this place I called home. Since that weekend, I've been in a continuous state of appreciation and gratitude for everything that I have in my life, every second of the day.

This was my new station in life. What I didn't realize after what changed in me at that weekend at Roberto's, was how much space I was going to give other people to be themselves when they were around me. I observed I no longer needed to control my environment in order to feel safe around others. Before, I had fixed perceptions and ideas of how things needed to look and be.

The next morning, I woke up and worked on the four postures that Roberto had given me to work on and that night I went and taught a women's group class at De Anza Cove in San Diego that was part of my fitness business. I had created this class as a safe space for women to work out and build sisterhood, and not feel like they were being ogled by men. It was a place where women could go and get a great workout.

Every Wednesday I would show up with a plan for their

workout, but that night things changed. I said to them, "Listen. I want you to warm up, but I want you to do what you want to do for a warm-up, and when you come back from your warm-up, if you want to walk, walk. If you want to run, run. If you want to stay here and jump rope for fifteen minutes, that's fine too. We're going to investigate what you want to do tonight, okay?" And they looked at me like confused dogs, with their heads cocked to the side.

I was consciously unaware in that moment that I was being different with them.

We got through the courses that night and I said to the group, "Listen, I saw this guy, he taught me a few things. We're going to be trying some of it here. All that other stuff that I used to be doing, I'm not interested in that anymore." I was surprised when it came out of my mouth.

At the time, my mind was retroactive. So even though I was in the experience, I didn't understand the impact of the experience until sometimes days, weeks, months, even years later. Because I had so much tension and stress in my body, brain, nervous system, organs, and channels, by the time an experience moved through my entire physical, mental, emotional, and spiritual body and came back into my psychological body, there was a lot of lag time. I didn't understand that my mind worked retroactively until it didn't.

I said, "Look, I got a buddy of mine who I used to be in the SEAL teams with, he's taught a couple of my courses here for you when I've been out of town traveling. If you want that kind of training, I'll give you his number. You can train with him." Some of the women left. Some of the women stayed.

Halfway through my drive home it hit me: I was different. I called Roberto when I got home.

"Dude, what happened? I'm not experiencing my life the same way."

He started laughing his ass off and then he told me, "Listen, as you take out tension, the person who you really are moves forward into your reality."

I was well on my way back to the self.

COMING BACK TO ME

Every day when I got down on the floor and worked on removing tension from myself, the real me began to emerge and the false self began to fall away. This process impacted the way I slept, the way I ate, even the movies I was attracted to. It impacted the books that I wanted to read, the events that I wanted to go to and experience. It affected everyone in my relationships and every single aspect of my life.

In less than two and a half months of doing this work on myself, I went from having people expressing how intense I was to talking about how peaceful and impactful my energy is. Strangers would stop me in the grocery store and literally tell me that my energy was incredible and beautiful, which to me was quite a shock. People's perception of me was based on how much tension I was holding. In my mind at that time, it was a little crazy.

I was floored. I knew that I was well on my way to regaining my health, but I didn't understand how that affected others. I later came to understand that I was doing more than creating health, I was dismantling my fear states and the false strength and armor I had used to keep myself protected throughout my life—from the Milton Hershey School to the SEAL team. People could subconsciously feel that I had changed, because the present is present. When your mind and body stop circulating fear that uses strategies based in separation consciousness to keep people away from your deepest emotional core wounds, you become vulnerable and allow others to connect to who it is you are underneath your pain, your confusion, your anger, your anxiety, and your fear. You become present and open to receive what the moment has to offer. You literally step into the receptive mode because you no longer operate from a place of fear. Emotionally, you're willing to risk connecting to others in your authenticity.

That first year was amazing. I built quality relationships with people and these people were focused on the same thing; the removal of tension from the body. Suddenly I was in this community of people that were being emotionally honest, open, authentic, generous, kind, compassionate, understanding, accepting, forgiving, devoted, loyal, fun, and funny.

When I was in Milton Hershey School and in the SEAL teams, the preferred form of relating was through sarcasm and stoicism. Now I was surrounded by people whose primary way of relating was through humor and vulnerability.

I was high on life every day. Often I would pinch myself and say, "Really? Is this my life now? How did this happen?"

There was so much change and the only thing I did was remove stress, tension, and distortion. And there was so much palpable and observable change that I could see within myself, and the unsolicited feedback I got from others confirmed how important the changes I was making really were. Really? That's it? You must be kidding me. How could it be that easy? Well, I was sure happy it was that easy. The truth is, there's no substitute. Either you're stressed, tense, and distorted, or you're not. If you are, you need to pull down the wall right now, get vulnerable, and ask for help. Whether you realize it or not now, the last few years of your life you are going to suffer and suffer and suffer and suffer and suffer and suffer and suffer. So, great! Live for the moment, yet at the end of the day, everybody who chooses to ignore all the flashing road signs pays the piper. I was lucky to pay the piper in my thirties, rather than my seventies and eighties. It was simple: relieve the stress, pull out the tension, dump the distortion, and who you really are underneath will emerge into effortless Being.

Keep lobbing in more stress, keep accumulating more tension and more distortion, and you know what you're going to get? You're going to get further, further, and further away from yourself and you're going to be operating at low-functioning behaviors (doing) versus high-functioning behaviors (being). What it really comes down to is this: do you want to do, or do you want to be?

At the end of the day, stress, tension, and distortion add up, and they cause separation from the authentic self. It's a formula that's equally as important to $E=mc^2$. Weakness precedes stress, stress precedes tension, tension precedes distortion. What exactly is weakness? When you use a coping strategy to relate to yourself or others, you're accessing your inauthenticity. Even if this coping strategy has led to your success in the world, you've still been using it to avoid punishment, rejection, humiliation, or any physical, mental, emotional, energetic, or psychic violence. Despite any of your success, that inauthenticity weakens you because you're consciously making the choice *not* to be you. The only way to be strong and connected is to express who you are authentically. Inauthenticity weakens absolutely. If you understand that, then you have a shot at getting out of the hell you're in. The majority of you don't have any idea you're in hell. That's what needs to be stated clearly. There isn't a human being on the planet who doesn't have a minimum of seven layers of generational stress, tension, and distortion, manifested as fear, anxiety, anger, and self-righteousness.

In life, we've been taught that the things outside ourselves have greater value than what is within. The philosophies, techniques, and methods contained within this book help you to uncover and find what's always been within: the true self.

About six to seven weeks into applying the stretching technique I learned from Roberto, I visited a couple of lifelong friends at Jeff Whitney's house. One of them was a woman named Lisa Shockley. As soon as I walked into the room, she looked at me and said, "Oh my god, Christopher, whatever you're doing, keep doing it, because you're almost back."

I had to take a step back for a second. What was she

talking about? I realized I had no idea what she was talking about until she brought up Homecoming at Milton Hershey School the previous year. I remember I had talked to a bunch of people that day and they all kept getting up and leaving the conversation. I thought it was odd, but never said anything. Lisa was one of the people who left the conversation abruptly, so I asked her why. She said, "When you came back to Homecoming, I knew that that little boy that I grew up with wasn't the same person. And I thought to myself, what happened to you? You were talking to me and saying f--k this and f--k that, and how the f--k and where the f--k and who the f--k. I never heard so many curse words inside of a five-minute conversation in my entire life. The energy coming through you was very toxic."

The most shocking part to me was that I didn't even realize that I had changed. I didn't know I was a person who cursed a lot. I had no clue my language had become offensive, hurtful, and toxic. I was unaware I was no longer being received as that sweet boy from Milton Hershey School, yet I could see it now. I could see how it happened. I could feel every step of separation from my true, authentic self.

All the stress, tension, and distortion builds little by little. Every day it comes into the body in such small increments that you don't realize it's happening and then one day you've completely changed. It's impacted the way you breathe, think, emote, sleep, feed, care for yourself, and all the ways in which you move through the world.

It's like an auto mechanic. He gets out of high school, goes to mechanic school for two years, and starts working on cars. He's constantly bending over and trying to hold his body up with the muscles in his low back. He thought he was normal until he went down one day to tie his shoes and ended up on a spine board, and now lives in chronic agony. Stiffness, discomfort, loss, and pain are the last indicators something's wrong. Most people make the assumption those are the *first* indicators something's wrong, and therefore look to place a Band-Aid over their symptoms out of ignorance and lack of awareness. It lacks the ability to perceive there's a bigger problem at play. The simplicity in all this is laughable, once you truly understand the nature of being. Stress, tension, and distortion equal separation from self, in a relative sense.

I thought I was normal until that day Lisa told me I wasn't. Knowing that the stretches were working, I committed to working on them even harder. I had all the confirmation that I needed to dive as deep as humanly possible into this process.

The interesting thing about this story is that when Roberto did his initial assessment on me, he pointed out that my gallbladder channel was completely out of balance. When that channel is out of balance, a person will curse a lot. When Lisa brought up our conversation at Homecoming, she reconfirmed that there was truth to Chinese meridian theory.

In the philosophy of Chinese meridian theory, the body has twelve primary channels filled with *chi*, or energy. The Chinese deconstruct energy into twelve distinct and nuanced qualities. A balanced, healthy body has *chi* that flows in a constant unrestricted manner. Within the core of every muscle travels a particular quality of energy that corresponds to a certain state of being and relating in the inner world and outer life.

According to Chinese meridian theory, consciousness resides inside the body. As the body accumulates more stress, it weakens and tightens as compensation, which chokes off the natural flow of *chi* and consciousness. All yoga postures are designed as a complement to allow us to access deeper and greater levels of being. Each one of the stretching positions I learned from Roberto had a direct and definite impact on how lymph, blood, and energy moved through my body and changed the ways in which I related, thought, sensed, and emoted in my inner and outer worlds.

FINDING MY OWN PATH

After my mom died, many women stepped into my life as strong and amazing mother figures. They were honest and they held me accountable for what I was saying and doing and thinking, and how I was impacting the shared environment that we were co-creating in. When you go through something like SEAL training, you have instructors that are older than you, that know the landscape of a SEAL Team life. But none of them acts as a father figure to you because SEAL Teams are about building and establishing brotherhood. My biological father was never present in my life, and Roberto filled out an important role for me. As the masculine aspect of myself began to mature, I realized it was time to venture out on my own in terms of what personal transformation meant to me. There comes a day where every boy looks at his father and decides he's going to do things his own way. It took me two years and three months to mature to that state of readiness and have the realization that it was time to do my own thing and discover the truths within truth for myself.

Roberto was an amazing teacher and guide. He taught me how to prepare specific types of foods, he took me to grocery stores, he showed me how to buy the best foods for my journey, I started to understand what "organic" really meant. He spent an intense amount of time and energy helping me grow beyond my limitations. I would not have become the person that I am today without his help. He was beyond generous, and he was a complete pain in the ass. His dogmatic personality made it difficult to be around. He had an idea and an opinion about everything, and his perceptive filters were fixed at that point. And there was no shifting or changing this man's idea of reality. I'm a bit that way myself, so I could empathize easily with where he was at in his outward expression of himself. Because I grew up institutionalized at Milton Hershey School, there was a clear right and there was a clear wrong. Life at Milton Hershey School was black and white. It took an extremely courageous woman to get me to understand that magic is what happens in the gray areas of life.

Everyone has their own orientation of the truth, and you must give people the spaciousness to find it without trying to get them fixed on your own perceptual filters. I was now looking for my own truth. That truth would eventually become my North Star, my mission, my motivating force in life, which I call True Body Intelligence. Without intelligence, it is impossible to manipulate our environment. High levels of intelligence enable us to move forward as a culture and a race. If we lack understanding of each physical, mental, emotional, spiritual, energetic, and sexual aspect, it becomes impossible for us to navigate the challenges coming to us next.

THE GIFT OF HONESTY

The greatest gift in life is people that care enough to tell us how we're impacting them. Honesty pulls us out of whatever delusion we're living under. The truth will hurt a little bit, but it will give you the opportunity to look at yourself clearly. When you have a clear understanding, you can choose where to put your time, energy, and resources and find someone who can help you make a shift.

Honesty brings you out of the dark and into the light. It's like when your mom came in at 6:30 in the morning and turned on the lights to get you up and ready for school. In that first moment, the light hitting your eyes was somewhat painful, but then as you start waking up and embracing your day, the light of day becomes pleasurable.

When people withhold honesty, they rob you of the opportunity to shift out of states of being, sensing, relating, and emoting that are sabotaging your opportunity to experience what it is that you want to experience at the deepest and the highest levels. With honesty, you have an opportunity to guide yourself towards inner freedom. Without honesty, you have no way of getting out of your own way. This is why it's best to surround yourself with people who care enough to tell you the things you don't want to hear. They will hold you accountable for how you're impacting them.

There are two versions of honesty. There's the inner honesty and the outer honesty. One's ability to allow others outside of them in on how they're feeling about them is outer honesty. Inner honesty is your ability to let you in on yourself and how you're feeling about how this dynamic, this situation, this person, this opportunity is impacting you. Some people are good at being honest with others, and some people are really good with being honest with themselves. Some people feel more comfortable being honest with themselves but they don't feel comfortable letting other people in on how they're feeling about them, because they want to avoid the punishment, rejection, humiliation, violence, and the feelings of separation that come along with living an honest, authentic, self-expressive life.

With the tools Roberto provided me, I could attain freedom from the inside out. I could work on myself in my own timing, and I could put as much effort and time and energy in as I wanted, or I could put in less if that's what felt correct for me in those moments. For me, the challenge with most wellness systems is that there's a patient and there's a practitioner, which creates some level of dependency and co-dependency. You have to rely on another person's skillset, passion, and ability to access unconditional love for themselves and their connection to their version of the creator. Even though Roberto did things and acted in certain ways that were counter to my ethics, I held him in high regard because he did what he said and he said what he was going to do. He underpromised and overdelivered.

The day that Lisa Shockley said I was almost back to the person she knew as a young adult, I knew it was time to find my own orientation to this work. De-stressing and de-tensing are valuable, and the techniques I learned from Roberto were great, but it was time for me to go on the real journey, which was figuring out how I wanted to work with myself and others.

I had a different vantage point from Roberto. He operated under the belief that he was the creator and he desperately wanted continuous credit for every good thing that manifested in your life. I believe that no one can be a true creator on their own and that we are all co-creators. Everything that exists is a process of co-creation. We are all co-creators with God, vessels for inspiration. To make dinner, you need knives, a cutting board, pots, pans, and a stove. A bird lands on a branch, eats a seed, flies away. A few hours later, the bird poops. That excrement falls to the ground and nourishes the soil, and the grass begins to grow.

Everything is a process of co-creation, and everything in life is recycled. There's never any more, and there's never any less. Nothing can ever be destroyed, it can only change form.

PUTTING IT TO THE TEST

Going through de-stressing and de-tensing and developing True Body Intelligence helped me understand the process of true transformation. De-stressing and de-tensing techniques I learned made so much sense because they were based on logic, but it was also based on data that Roberto had gathered for a few decades. From his own orientation to truth, he put it to the test.

When I separated from Roberto, I had to put my own work to the test. I needed to come up with my own orientation and understanding of the value of de-stressing and de-tensing. I needed to determine for myself what was the implicit order to follow in order to take someone through a true transformational process.

As a teacher, as a guide, as a coach, and as a friend, my focus and intention has always been to listen first. Gather the data, and respond and initiate appropriately. What I tell my students all the time is this: If you call me up seven years from now and you're still doing the work the way you learned it from me, I have failed you miserably. What works for me works for me when I work with people. If you choose to become a parrot, what you give up is the opportunity to discover who you are. Some parrots can be really great parrots. Yet, if you're a monkey pretending to be a parrot, you're a failure. All the great wisdom teachers have pointed out that great men find the courage to do things their own way.

If you're a lion, you need to be a lion. If your circumstances that you were reared under caused you to take on the characteristics of a zebra to keep you safe because the environment was chaotic and violent, then your strategy was an effective strategy to adopt. At some point, your strategy is going to become your own worst enemy. Once you get into your 30s, 40s, and 50s, those fear-based strategies you're employing are only going to cause you to feel depressed, alone, confused, anxious, angry, self-righteous, and separate.

Every animal in the jungle is going to think the lion is crazy if he's out hanging out with a bunch of giraffes and eating coconuts. They're going to be like, "Look at that crazy-ass lion. He thinks he's a giraffe!" If you had to pretend to be a giraffe because your circumstances were violent and unpredictable when you were younger, then that's okay. But if you're really a lion, at some point you have to find the courage to take off the giraffe costume and be honest with everyone in your environment. That's going to take a really big set of balls, because going along for the ride is easy.

I needed to find my own orientation in order to be effective in the world; I had to take ownership of who I was becoming. In order for me to take ownership of that, I had to walk away from the person who had become my teacher. I had to get my own unique sense and learn my own orientation to all things.

Who am I in relationship to money? Who am I in relationship to food? Who am I in relationship to religion? Who am I in relationship to nature? Who am I in relationship to sexuality? Who am I in relationship to knowledge? Who am I in relationship to community? Who am I in relationship to freedom? Who am I in relationship to creativity? Who am I in relationship to liberty? Who am I in relationship to boundaries? Who am I in relationship to principles? Who am I in relationship to ethics? Who am I in relationship to morals? Who am I in relationship to truth? Who am I in relationship to forgiveness? And lastly and most importantly, who am I in relationship to love?

Finding love is an impossibility without discovering freedom first.

MOVING ON FROM ROBERTO TO TRUE BODY INTELLIGENCE

True Body Intelligence is an opportunity to change and transform that which is inevitable. There will never be any more or any less energy in your body, it only matters whether or not you have access to it. Every bit of stress, every bit of tension, every bit of distortion that's in your body interrupts and encumbers the natural flow of *chi* and consciousness from top to bottom, from back to front, from left to right, from in to out. The ability to find someone who will gift you the opportunity to take responsibility for what you co-created when you were unconscious and disjointed and asleep is a gift in and of itself.

It was difficult for me to tell Roberto what I had learned on my own, because I didn't want to hurt his feelings. I avoided confrontation because he had given me so much. Now that I'm older, I realize that not telling him was more cruel, because I never gave him the opportunity to change and to speak for himself. The honesty I value the most from others is the thing that I withheld the most from him.

He was honest with me. He told me all things I didn't want to hear, and in the end, I didn't ante up that way for him. I bowed out with what I thought was grace, but it wasn't gracious. Gracious would've been me telling him the truth.

In the end, the person who's the most honest is the person that's the most vulnerable. Every guru I've ever met has had a horrific amount of trauma. And Roberto was no different. Children who are traumatized lose the ability to be authentically vulnerable and they manipulate through ck, and violence.

If Roberto had told me that he wanted to learn why I had such rapid changes from the stretches for his own desires, wants, and needs, and to become more successful, I would have agreed because everything would've started from a place of honesty. When I understand the why behind someone's motivation, I can make the personal choice whether or not to participate.

Once people realize that they are participating in something that they don't want to participate in, then the relationship is over. And if you lack the ability to communicate authentically and honestly, then you're screwed.

Roberto is a highly intelligent human being. Intelligence is one's ability to manipulate their environment to produce the result that they want. Roberto manipulated his environment. It was inhumane in the sense that it never informed me of the real reasons why he wanted to participate and help me. I was always under the illusion that he was being so incredibly generous, but he had an ulterior motive. He wasn't upfront that he needed me as much as I needed him. In relationships, if you manipulate without giving the real level of information to the other person, eventually they'll feel excluded regardless of how wonderful the experience has been. If they feel at some point that you've been dishonest with them, they're going to feel like everything that they gained from you is terrible anyway.

Anyone can self-express, but finding the courage to communicate clearly while considering where the other person is in real space and time, in terms of their development, and how they're going to process that information and take it in and how it may potentially impact their relationship, that is an ascended level of relating. Clear communication is the ascended path to establishing inner and outer peace. In my relationship with Roberto, there was no clear communication, there was only agenda-driven self-expression. I love to be around people who authentically self-express. There is a certain amount of entertainment value, but what I've discovered over time is that I feel emotionally safe around people who have the ability to communicate clearly their real feelings, thoughts, and intentions.

CHAPTER 3

THE LEARNING PROCESS

In 1999, I didn't know anything about juicing and I'd never even heard the word yoga, but after that one session with my buddy, Jeff Higgs, I decided to try it. I showed up at a heated yoga class that smelled awful from the moment I stepped through the door. The teacher immediately called me out in front of the forty other students. She said, "Look what we got here, kids, we got somebody with muscles."

Of course, the whole room was surrounded by mirrors and everyone stared at me. I thought, "Who is this lady picking on me because I have muscles?" but then I thought, maybe these muscles are a problem. The egocentric part of me wanted to slam her on the ground, but the other part of me knew that there was something to what she was saying, so I stuck around the class for a while.

I was stiff, but when I left, I felt incredible. Jeff and I continued yoga. At the same time, I started receiving deep tissue massage, and each week I started to feel a little better. For so long I was in pain, but my goal and my need to get the golden trophy was so big that I kept overriding my body's systems that were on red alert going, *Christopher stop. Christopher stop. Christopher stop.*

From here I met James Bulger and added Hellerwork to my regimen. Then, my biggest lesson came in 2000 when I was in my car accident. I woke up the next morning with a deep, intense throb in the middle of my hip, and no matter what I did, I could never get away from the discomfort. The insurance company provided resources for me to get holistic treatments, so I did the Egoscue Method, Hellerwork, deep tissue massage, yoga, plus acupuncture. At this point, when I wasn't working with others, I was working on myself. At the time, I was quite happy with the changes because I didn't know that you could get instantaneous, permanent change, and I stayed focused on the methods I was learning from the holistic practitioners.

In comparison, after I worked with Roberto and I got that instantaneous permanent change that I was looking for,

I was lit up from the inside out. I received an incredible, unique education from Roberto. The real education came from doing the work he taught me on myself, which, at the time, he called stretches. I would go home and spend five to six hours a day working through these positions. While I was in those positions, I began to understand how to work with each part of my body, and I could feel all the disjointedness from top to bottom, back to front, left to right, inside to outside. I began to understand interconnectedness from the inside out. After doing something with my upper body, I would then go back to doing something with my lower body, and I could feel how much more open my lower body was because of what I did to my upper body and vice versa.

This is when I learned the interconnectedness of top to bottom, back to front, in to out, left to right. I realized that if the outside of my left was short and tight then the inside of my right was short and tight as well, so I could start to feel all the bilateral malformations. It was shocking to discover how much stress and tension were twisting my structural form as well as my emotional availability, from the inside out.

Three months into de-stressing and de-tensing, I decided to study with a guy named Dennis Paulsen. I read his book and went on a fifty-three day fast, which turned out to be extremely educational. This was a big learning tool because at that time I didn't understand that my body stored tons of toxicity in its organs. With the fast, I had an opportunity to rid myself of a majority of the toxins I had accumulated from thirty-three years and three months of unconscious living.

I didn't take in any solid food. The only thing I did was drink hot teas, vegetable broth, and fresh juice. What I learned is that people are full of parasites. We may see that stuff in TV shows and think there's nothing like that in our bodies, but one day I dumped twenty-five large parasites. That was a real wake up call. I now understood that there were things going on inside of the body that I had no clue about. This experience then caused me to investigate further into how to care for my entire body and take responsibility for my choices in foods. I completely altered the way in which I moved through the world.

Once I decided to go out on my own and discover the work and my process of true transformation, even bigger changes occurred. Me, my brother Marcus Riggleman, and my two buddies Nic and Kyle Shinners started to work together on each other using the basic techniques we learned and began enhancing them by implementing isometric and concentric contractions to balance out all the excessive over-stretching we had learned from Roberto. In no time, our bodies began to step back into balance. Nic created what we called at the time a stretching board that allowed the person being stretched to access maximal force, resistance, and connection, and his genius allowed us to change ten times faster than what was then humanly possible.

Nic and I began working on each other for three to four hours at a time, a minimum of three days a week, for a year and a half straight. Up until that time, I hadn't yet had a cathartic experience with the stretching, and then suddenly, about a year in, we were working intensely on removing tension from my lateral hamstring, and emotionally I could feel all these intense feelings of separation well up into my breath and my eyes, and I lost it. I cried and cried and cried. Emotionally, Nic had no idea what to do, which was OK. He literally didn't understand how to support anybody emotionally, yet he gave me the space I needed, and I literally laid there on the floor for three hours, heaving, sighing, and crying. Each heave, each sigh, and each tear being released softened my heart to a level that I remembered accessing before Mrs. Baskerfield put my hands on the gas stove. I was truly stepping back into who I would have become had I not been traumatized by that event. Consciously, I knew that the body stores emotions, but this was the first time I'd experienced it from the inside out. When you heave and cry that hard from a physical release and not because something happened in the moment, it's quite a different experience. My heart was lighter, and my original childhood trauma was being evacuated. No matter how hard or how much I attempted to hold back my tears, it was an unstoppable force of action. I no longer had the need to control my environment, myself, or anyone else in order to feel safe and present.

Once I got done, and learned all I could with my own body, I started working with people. This is when I began to see and understand the patterns in people's bodies, their energy fields, and their emotions. It was during this time I decided to get a formal education in Chinese medicine.

In May 2005, I enrolled at The Pacific College of Chinese Medicine. I had a general understanding of de-stressing and de-tensing, but I needed to go deeper. I wanted to know where and how this information was originally obtained. I needed formal education on the subject so that I could teach it to others. I began to learn the different qualities of *chi* and energy and was able to understand why the stretches I had done with Roberto and created on my own were working. In Chinese medicine, energy worked in opposites. There was hot and cold, stagnant and flowing, excessive and deficient. Pain could then be described as dull and achy or fixed and stabbing.

All I knew before was that the goal of the stretches was to eliminate tension, what I now understood was that the reason they worked is that their real goal was to balance the chi. In Chinese medicine, there is an age-old saying, "Where there is pain there is no flow; where there is no flow, pain is sure to follow."

SEEING THE LIGHT

After my first semester at The Pacific College, I took a trip to Mount Shasta. I had just come down the mountain after snowboarding for four hard hours. I was looking outside the back window off the porch, and suddenly I saw this piece of wood, and around the piece of wood was this enormous green aura, and I thought, "Am I crazy? Did I just make this stuff up in my head?" I closed my eyes, opened them back up, and it was still there. I did that repeatedly for fifteen minutes.

In Chinese medicine, they have a theory called the five elements theory. In the five elements theory, each organ is related to a specific element, and each element is related to a specific color. The color of the element of wood, and the two organs associated with it—the gallbladder and the liver—emit the color green.

That day, the green around the wood was the most beautiful green I'd ever seen. The aura was a wake-up call for me and it was something I was able to see from then on.

From that moment forward, when people came to see me

to start de-tensing and de-stressing, I could see a small aura around them, and I was able to relate the color of the aura to where their state of inner wellbeing was. As they began to implement the de-stressing and de-tensing techniques I taught them, their aura started to become whiter and brighter with each succeeding session.

Not only were others changing around me, but so was I. The more integrated I became, from the inside out, top to bottom, back to front, in to out, and the more I got my energy in alignment, the easier it was for me to not only see these types of phenomena but also learn these types of things from the inside out.

Studying Chinese medicine taught me the nomenclature and valuable information, but when I received acupuncture every day, I felt a real shift in my energy. In Chinese medicine, the focus is dissolving stagnation, to remove the energy that stops your organs and consciousness from functioning at a high capacity.

After studying Chinese medicine, in 2007 I decided to go to the University Healing Dao. I flew to Thailand and started studying. I learned about healing sounds, the inner smile, and the microcosmic orbit, and circulating energy between your Ren and your Du channels. I then went on what's called the Dark Room Retreat, and in the dark room retreat I was in complete darkness for twenty-eight days. There was not one photon of light, and my body went into whole different states of seeing, feeling, emoting, thinking, meditating, expanding, and integrating.

During the first three days in the dark room my body basically slept. I woke up. I ate a little food. I went back to sleep. I woke up. I ate a lot of food. I went back to sleep. I woke up, I ate, and I went back to sleep.

By day four when I woke up, I had tons and tons of energy. The dark room process and adjusting to a light-free atmosphere caused my body to release a maximal amount of melatonin into my blood. Once the release of melatonin reached its maximal saturation point, my pineal gland began releasing a neurotransmitter called pynomine into my bloodstream. Once that reached its maximal saturation point, my brain began releasing the first of two spiritual molecules—OM5E. After OM5E reached its maximal saturation point, I began a twenty-four-hour-a-day release of DMT. After DMT reached its maximal saturation point, I began a twenty-four-hour-a-day DMT journey for three and a half weeks.

My third eye was completely open. While I was sitting and listening and following the meditations, mantras, and the physical Taoist practices, I could simultaneously use my third eye to peer into a completely different dimension.

The basic practices in the dark room were how to be the inner smile, the six healing sounds, and the microcosmic orbit. During that twenty-eight-day process, I learned to sleep and get all the rest that my body needed. As you can imagine, SEAL trainings, and training for the Olympic trials and medical school, used up an intense amount of my energetic reserve. I was beginning to feel alive again in a way that was new and multidimensional.

One of the things that still boggles my mind today and is quite interesting about the dark room process was that there were about sixty people in this dark room, all moving in and around and about, and at no time during that twenty-eight days did I bump into another human being. I bumped into a few walls, which was kind of funny at that time. Each participant had their individual space for their yoga mat, where they would go through the dark room training. Five times a day for twenty-eight days, I ended up exactly where I needed to be without any outer visual input. One week I used sound; another week I used smell. The final week I used my sense of energy. I now understood how people could get around in the outer world, being completely blind and completely OK with it. All my senses were heightened at a level that 99.9 percent of all human beings who've ever lived will never, ever reach. I feel more than fortunate to have had that experience.

During that time, by the fifth day, I walked through the

door of all wonder, and I saw and experienced things for the next twenty-three days that you only feel and see in movies. I saw my past lives; I saw my future lives. I saw my purpose laid out for me in this life. I could write a 300-page novel on that experience alone, and yet I won't because that experience is really meant for those who truly desire to experience human potential at its greatest level.

After the darkroom retreat, the next level of education I got was when I decided to journey to Iceland. There I started studying Native American mysticism and sweat lodges. Every few weeks I would go to a Native American-designed sweat lodge in Iceland, and that's where I began to understand the deep impact of fire and water, hot and cold. Up at 66° North, there are experiences available to you that you simply will never find anywhere else.

At the Native American-designed sweat lodge, they did specific rounds based on the elements and the four cardinal directions. The first round might be air, then water, then fire, and so on. In my fifth round during this experience, they sang a very special Native American song and the heat had reached its maximum. Whether my eyes were open or closed, I saw the same thing: a movie screen directly in front of me and for fifteen minutes straight, women's faces would appear, move toward me, and then disappear. From their outfits and my study in Icelandic history, I could tell these women were from the 1300s and 1600s.

As you can imagine, seeing that kind of thing might freak you out. Yet the last few years of experiences had prepared me to maintain my center while connecting to each one of these souls. I realized I was helping them to transition back to the light. What a beautiful, powerful, and impactful experience. Seeing those faces was a wild, beautiful, and powerfully impactful experience. Looking back keeps me motivated to continue to understand and grow beyond my own inner limitations.

Throughout my learning, every couple of months I would go through a cleansing process. I kept de-stressing, de-tensing, and de-distorting, which continued to eliminate confusion and illusions, helping me to continue to keep becoming less dis-integrated and more present as I reintegrated the broken, disjointed aspects of myself back into the whole. After some time, I returned home from Iceland and began to study sacred geometry and the impact of intention, form, and magnetism on energetic intelligence and spiritual development. I began to feel and see the full impact of products designed to transmute low-functioning waveforms into high-functioning energy fields. The intention for the creation of these products was simply to transmute the negative back into the positive.

The biggest lesson for me in all this work was that, although I valued educating myself, it wasn't up to me to figure it all out. I could allow my intuition to guide me, and I could allow my intention to be the driving force for what I attracted to myself. I was shifting from the masculine, problem-solving initiator into the feminine, receptive, intuitive being that I had the potential to be.

Along the way, I've worked with many different niches and demographics. I've worked with billionaires and the poorest of the poor. I've worked with incredibly smart people and people who have average or below-average intelligence. I've worked with people who have high levels of emotional intelligence and those with very low levels of emotional, social intelligence.

In the end, I learned that there's no substitute for de-stressing and de-tensing and de-distorting. There's no substitute for meditation, acupuncture, breath work, and de-distortion. You could eat all the best foods in the world, but if your body is full of stress, tension, and distortion, you'll only absorb a small amount of those nutrients. An extremely limiting belief is believing that eating healthy means you're healthy. To be honest with you, it's complete nonsense. Stress and your orientation to stress are a greater determiner of health than anything else.

My unique education allowed me to discover the

implicate order to follow in order to attain a high level of wellbeing. I am clear on what's good for what, and through diligent concerted effort, I've learned the hard way the limitations of every single one of these systems. The great learning and teaching have been that there's no substitute for any one of these systems, and if you're going to focus on your health and wellness, you have to be focused on every one of these aspects. You have to focus on developing your physical, mental, emotional, environmental, and spiritual intelligence. You must focus a bit of your time, energy, and resources on caring for yourself. You need to focus a bit of your time and energy on structural integration. You need to focus a bit of your time and energy on meditation. You should focus a bit of your energy on psychological and emotional development. Lastly, you need to focus an intense amount of time, energy, and resources on de-stressing and de-tensing if you're ever going to reach even close to your individual human potential that lies within your own innate genius. It's all a process.

THE RESULT

I've been devoted and dedicated for seventeen years without ever taking my eye off the ball. The first seven years I was incredibly focused on the density and impact of stress and tension on the human body and all the individual energetic systems. From 2008 on, I focused on the brain and the nervous system, and understanding how energy moves through, in, and out of the body, and how to communicate clearly by talking to the body and giving it permission to heal itself in its own timing.

This all caused me to create an entirely new body of work called Body of Light. Within Body of Light, there are activations, attunements, and what I call Clean Sweeps, where we sweep through all major systems and reintegrate all the places where negative and false projections about reality are disturbing the natural flow of energy, chi, and consciousness. Once your nervous system realizes it no longer needs to be loyal to low-functioning false interpretations about reality, you will feel a lightness and spaciousness inside of you and the desire to again explore discovering who you are in relationship to any one thing on this third-dimensional plane of projection, reflection, and manifestation. You can begin to see them as your self, and you can make incredible changes.

Balanced humans are the humans of the future. In order to attain balance, you must increase your physical, mental, emotional, spiritual, and environmental intelligence so that you're clear on the full impact that your conscious, unconscious, and subconscious choices are having on you from the inside out, top to bottom, back to front, in to out, and, lastly, from out to in. I am confident that Body of Light will help any human being seeking internal freedom and outer peace through self-reintegration at an extremely deep level.

I have spent the last seventeen years devoted to this path. I did this so that it wouldn't take people like you seventeen years to get to where I am today. Are you ready for instantaneous, permanent change? That's the real question, isn't it? Are you ready to feel and access inner freedom so that you may be in outer peace with the rest of the world, in, around, and about you?

CHAPTER 4

TWO CARS FROM
THE JUNKYARD

Most people have no idea who they really are. People
think they *are* whatever it is that they *do*. In my experience of men, they wear what they do as a badge of honor.
They'll say "Oh, I graduated from Harvard, *summa cum
laude*." Then that man finds a woman, or her family,
who holds him in high regard because of what he's done,
rather than who he BE (is). When you put that person
in that environment, and they're focused on receiving a
reward for what they do rather than being rewarded for
who they BE (are), eventually they'll fall because they
aren't focused on Being. Eventually the luster of what you
do wears away if you're an asshole behind closed doors.
Doing is only attractive for so long, and bringing attention
to your Doing is unattractive, yet Being is the only thing

that lasts forever. So the question begs: are you tired of your ego's need for incessant attention for what you do, or would you rather be respected for who you've become through this journey we call life?

When your focus is on doing, you shift out of the receptive mode and into the initiatory mode, which is an assertive mode. It is impossible to maintain a long-term, loving relationship if you're continuously in the initiatory mode. Vulnerability is the ascended quality because it shifts you emotionally and physically into the receptive mode. If you're someone who's endured any level of childhood stress, your focus is on doing, rather than being. And your awareness subconsciously and unconsciously is to avoid punishment, rejection, humiliation, and violence. Therefore, you keep yourself busy in Doing. What I discovered in SEAL training is that it's easy to hit a static target, and it's extremely difficult to hit a moving target. When you're being, you're receptive, allowing life to present itself to you. When you're continuously initiating to avoid punishment, rejection, humiliation, and violence, life is running away from you. In order to focus on being, you have to be in the receptive mode, meaning you have to attain a certain level of vulnerability and openness in your body, in your energy, in your emotions, and in your mind. Yet that's the last thing most of us feel comfortable being: vulnerable. We attempt to control our nt so that we're able to receive in the specific way that matches the tiny little box that we're operating out of. Even then we're curating what we want to receive and we're not openly receiving what life is presenting to us through vulnerability, openness, peacefulness, and inner freedom. When people push up against the places you haven't dealt with, the first thing you do is hop right back into your tiny, little box or force them to leave their box and join you in yours.

True Body Intelligence is about creating a pattern interrupt and breaking down the density and dismantling the stress that keeps those walls and boxes fixed, unmovable, and rigid. When you finally decide to break down those walls, you suddenly have the experience, for the first time in your life, of Being. Doing suddenly seems ridiculous and nonsensical. Being has great inner value. Doing has some outer value. It's more important to Be open-minded than it is to do research. It's more important to Be in a state of inner freedom than it is to go on vacation. It's more important to Be in a state of peacefulness than it is to sacrifice yourself to maintain relationships with others.

Achieving as a goal is an empty experience. Take a man who values title, status, and resources over vulnerability, honesty, and openness. He believes that his value comes from what he does, and so should be rewarded heavily for doing. None of his attention has gone into developing his BEing. After a while, his wife will begin to lose interest, and she will leave him because of his lack of vulnerability, sensitivity, openness, and inner and outer honesty. For weeks on end, his mind will continue to spin out on this idea: how could she do this to him after all he's DONE for her? Now, hopefully, he gets to the ascended state of understanding where he takes a left turn and trades down from BEing into doing. No amount of doing is a substitute for BEing. Now he shifts into the position from the provider and protector to the martyr, and he clings desperately to his resources as a justification and rationalization for his separation from self. The judge rewards the wife 50 percent or more of what's been accumulated since their marriage, and he wakes up and he's pissed and angry and as resentful as any good martyr could be. In his mind, he claims he did all this work and believes she took all his money. But the truth is, she tied her wagon to a man who shifted from Being and focused on doing and made the outer world of greater importance than discovering who he really is.

It doesn't matter how wealthy, successful, or famous you are, if you do not understand that who you are is separate from what you do, you're going to be miserable, and you'll do everything you can do to numb out from ever having to feel your separation from your authentic self. When you place a greater value on what you do rather than who you are, you are heading directly towards misery because whatever it is you do, you will eventually have to stop doing. And when you don't do that anymore, who is left in the aftermath? You don't have a clue, because you've never focused on who you are Being. We are human Beings, rather than human Doers. I've seen athletes who leave the game and end up selling drugs or having sex with teens because they've bought into their own false identity. I've watched the rich and the famous who've lost all their money and have no idea what to do next, simply because they never placed any value on Being. Being what? Being kind, being generous, being compassionate, being open, being honest, being powerful, being sweet, being devoted, being loyal, being gentle, being considerate, being free, and being love.

Once you begin de-stressing, de-tensing, and de-toxing, the new inner levels of vitality will cause you to look everywhere you can to find ways to remove and dismantle greater levels of stress, tension, and distortion that have been corrupting your experience of yourself, so that you can begin to get in touch with who it is you are underneath all the stress, tension, and distortion you've been accumulating since the moment the sperm penetrated the ovum. First you must understand the internal forces, the genetic and epigenetic markers that have caused you to separate yourself from your own unique authenticity and orientation towards intelligence, love, and light.

The sources of discomfort and emotional and psychological disintegration we all inherited go far back into each of our unique genetic histories. Stress, tension, and distortion are not something that appears simply because of our life experiences. Unless it is dealt with, it is passed down from generation to generation. Part of my pain began in the womb when my mother was forced to hide my birth because my father was of mixed race. While not everything is caused by racial relations, everything does begin when your father and mother come together. They each bring their own pains and psychological discomforts to the creation of their child. Their inner deficiencies become your inner deficiencies, and if there is not a pattern interrupt, your inner deficiencies will become your children's inner deficiencies. You'll pass your shortcomings to generation to generation to generation. Wouldn't it be more prudent to do the deep inner work and give your children the life they deserve?

Imagine that your mom and dad went to a junkyard. They each picked out a car, cut it in half, and welded those two halves together, then gave you that "Franken-car" and tried to convince you when you were a teenager that they gave you a brand-new car, right off the dealership's lot. The car is analogous to your body. It may look brand new and appear perfect from the outside, but it is carrying the weight of not only your parents' interactions with the world, but the interactions of their parents and the parents of those parents and so on, for a minimum of four to seven generations.

I remember my tenth-grade religious studies teacher, Mr. Cook, saying, "The sins of your forefathers will be revisited for four to seven generations." At the time, I wondered what he meant, yet of all the things I learned in school, it's the only thing I remember. It crystallized in my mind that day and took me on a sixteen-year journey of living out, day after day, night after night, the sins of my forefathers, meaning the shortcomings of my parents, and their parents, and their parents, and *their* parents. Shortcomings can be easily understood as a lack of either physical, mental, emotional, spiritual, spatial, and environmental intelligence. It took me on a sixteen-year journey. On the seventeenth year, I started with Roberto. Two days into my seventeenth year, I came to understand exactly what Mr. Cook meant when he said, "The sins of your forefathers will be revisited for four to seven generations." Physically, mentally, emotionally, and spiritually, I was devolving. The reflection of my life staring back at me could no longer be ignored. Anxiety replaced excitement. Frustration replaced freedom. Anger replaced love. Fear replaced fearlessness. Self-righteousness stood in place of righteous behavior, relative to self, family, community, culture, and planet.

That pile of junk you're moving around in is the "car" that

was handed down to you and has been in your family for a minimum of four to seven generations. Only a really talented mechanic could get it operational and safe to drive. Your parents' inner deficiencies have been passed along to you. That might mean soft teeth, a weak heart, poor vision, or a propensity for abuse or limiting financial beliefs. You might not even know what those limitations are until something goes tragically wrong. Your father could be unaware of that weak heart until he suddenly suffers a fatal heart attack. You may have anxiety that stems from an experience your great grandmother had. Every time your parents shut you down, every time your parents cut you off, every time your parents yell at you, every time they try to manipulate you, every time they try to use fear-based strategies to control you, that energy is coming from somewhere in their past or your ancestors' past.

Epigenetics is what's passed down from generation to generation in terms of behaviors, mood, feelings, and function. These conditions are called "epigenetic markers." These markers are often seen in children who are sexually abused. Tragedies are passed down from generation to generation until they are changed. It's difficult for these families to get out of the mess because although it may appear so, the tragic force isn't external, it is internal.

Whatever is going on inside of you is what you attract to you.

Suppose you had two children. One was born from a king and a queen and the other was born from peasant stock. The peasant's parents have run on survival strategies whereas the prince's parents have run on thriving strategies. One is love-based, one is fear-based. One feels entitled to experience whatever he or she desires in the world, and the other continues to question whether or not he or she is worthy to have such experiences. Let's say we switch the children at birth. The prince goes with the peasants and the peasant child goes with the royal family. You might think these kids will grow up differently because of their new circumstances, however, their past will follow them. The kid living with the poor family will still be treated like a prince because that's what his epigenetic markers dictate. The poor kid living in the castle may be handed the kingdom but will lose it because he has all the limiting beliefs that get expressed in survival-based thinking, feeling, and emoting. In a certain way, your epigenetics help become your identity.

A person's lifetime accumulated stress load is made up of their nature plus their nurture: the generational and the individual. Their nature is their genetics and the unresolved stress from previous generations. Nurture comes from the environment in which they grow, and this includes everything from birth and childrearing to the present: all the choices they've made throughout their lives, including all the choices they were driven to make by the previous generations.

The only way to change your markers and get out of the hell you're in is to take what's internally distorted and being expressed in your physical, mental, emotional, and energetic bodies and rewire your system from the inside out. Whatever is in you that's not you, corrupts you. That corruption limits you from experiencing the true you. At some point, everyone will discover what's actually going on underneath the hood. For many of us, myself included, that will happen in one's late twenties. As a Navy SEAL and someone who had always succeeded at everything I did, it came as a shock to me when I realized the body that I thought was a Porsche began to fall apart and look and feel and operate like a Ford Pinto.

When that happens, you have a choice to make: you can either take heartfelt action and choose to dismantle and dissolve through de-stressing, de-tensing, and de-distorting or you can ignore your disposition and retreat into distractions such as alcohol, nicotine, caffeine, recreational or pharmaceutical drugs, sex, work, or, the worst, exercise, which was the decision I made.

I used extreme exercise to run away from what was within. I kept thinking that the things holding me back were external forces, instead of realizing that they were internal distortions. I ignored my epigenetics until I could no longer move. The stiffness, discomfort, and pain kept attempting to bring my attention inward, and I only continued to focus my attention on outer goals and refused to take a look at my own limiting beliefs. If you choose to continue to ignore your body and all the signs and signals it's giving you, your true identity, you literally will grind yourself down to a halt.

WHATEVER IS IN THE BODY IS IN THE LIFE

I learned a lot of great information while studying the principles of Chinese medicine and Taoism. The universal practices they developed have given me the opportunity to understand that whatever is in my body is in my life, meaning whatever is in your life is also in your body. We live on a third-dimensional plane of projection and reflection expressed through generation after generation and manifestation.

What the Taoist masters figured out over time is that we have specific channels of energy that move from the organs out through the limbs. In the lower body, we have six channels and in the upper body, six channels. These twelve channels are called primary channels of energy, or "meridians," and are where our consciousness gets expressed. If an organ gets too hot, it's going to dump that excess heat down into the channel. If my heart is getting excessively hot, it will get expressed as fire in my emotions.

When we look at channels of energy and meridians,

each channel is connected to a specific world. What the Taoists figured out was that there are different types of constitutions. The masters who have done the research come from feminine cultures. Their belief system is that the feminine organs have all the function. The heart, for instance, pumps blood as its function. The pancreas creates digestive enzymes that the body needs to break down the food, so it has a function. The liver builds the blood and creates all the molecules for carbohydrates, proteins, and fat. It processes all that, so it has function.

The masculine organs, in terms of how the Taoists look at it, are just sacks that hold things. The bladder is a sack; it holds urine. The large intestine is a sack, it holds the bowel. The small intestine is a sack, it holds food. The gall bladder is a sack that holds bile. For the Taoists, the yin organs (feminine organs) have value, while the yang or masculine organs don't have any value because the Taoists don't value the holding of space. The masculine organs hold space for the feminine energies to function.

The Taoists look at the body in terms of hot or cold, excessive or deficient, yin or yang, masculine or feminine. This is how we all learn, simply through contrast. That's how they break things down. The way we apply this science that they've been gathering for thousands and thousands of years is to simply educate people about the impact of temperature on emotions.

Imagine your lover is in a state of fear as it relates to your relationship. If she has more cold in her kidneys than heat in her heart, she is going to withdraw and become unavailable by shutting down her ability to communicate her own innate fears that are being brought to the surface for review. But if she has more heat in her heart than she has cold in her kidneys, she's going to be in the attack mode. She's going to come after all the places where you're insecure, rather than admit her own insecurities. Fear in the kidneys translates to cold. Fear in the heart translates to heat.

What we want is to help people change their way of relating. People react based on how their body feels in that moment, how their brain and nervous system are processing stress. That means that they have no choice but to act and behave in a prescribed manner when a circumstance is delivered beyond their capacity to process emotionally. They have been hard-wired through their epigenetics and individually learned patterns of energy from childhood that are moving through their body and communicating in a unique, specific way. The way that they're communicating is relative to what they've accumulated in terms of their own states of fear that get expressed through anxiety, positions of self-righteousness, and anger.

Fear shifts all of us out of our natural human, spiritual states of being. And these fears express themselves as self-righteousness; conditional states of love, anger, and intense amounts of anxiety and disconnection; or an avoidance to having a very specific type of experience. Our natural base state for the heart—the physical body—is love, kindness, and compassion. The natural base state of the liver—the emotional body—is excitement. The natural base state of the spleen—the spiritual body—is righteousness, relative to self, family, community, culture, nation, and globe. The natural base state of the kidneys—the mental body—is fearlessness. Fear causes all of us to downshift from high-functioning states of being into low-functioning states of being. These are the natural states that we continuously move away from when we let our fears take control of us from the inside out.

FINDING THE NATURAL STATE

Fear lends itself to confusion. In that state of confusion is doubt, which prevents us from making the correct decision and ultimately keeps us from experiencing what it is we want to experience.

Suppose you're on a deserted island and need water. You might say, "There's a coconut in the tree." And then question, "What if I fall climbing the tree? I could die." You'll give yourself 110 reasons not to climb that tree. The next thing you know, you're dying because you can't get over enough of your fear to enable yourself to get the coconut and drink the fluid that ultimately will help you sustain your life.

If you're willing to move through your fears, be completely present, and take the correct action necessary to achieve what it is you want to experience, you will find that life is quite rewarding. If you do the inverse, you will find life to be quite defeating. And in so doing you will discover that whatever fears you're unwilling to move through actually capture you and steal your opportunity to connect to your authentic self.

People turn their TVs on to watch someone like LeBron James for two to three hours a day, two to three times a week for six months a year during a sports season. Why do they do it? Simple: LeBron is doing what he wants to do with his life and every day finds the courage to move through another layer of his own internal fears. That is something inspiring to observe. He does what feels natural to him, and he is encouraged by the world around him to keep being what it is he came here to be. And so, we reward him not only with our attention but also with giving him intense access to energy and resources.

Imagine that you come home every day and your mom tells you something positive about yourself. She gives you some positive feedback about who it is you are and what she recognizes as valuable in you to her. Every time that happens, your energy, your _chi,_ flows a little bit better. Now, imagine you had a twin who was separated at birth. He goes home to a household where his mother did the exact opposite thing. Every day, she pointed out one or several things that she believed he was doing wrong: "Your hair. It just looks terrible," says the negative mom. "You need to put a part in the middle, it looks better that way." She wants your twin to employ an unnatural state of relating for himself which compromises his ability to explore how he wants to present himself in terms of his looks. She's more focused on her feeling more comfortable about his presentation, which in turn makes her feel safe. Even though it looks as if she's looking out for him, she's really looking out for her.

Your twin's mother is expressing from an inorganic state of relating and being (conditional states of love), while your mother is coming from a natural state of being (unconditional states of love and kindness). All natural states of being create more flow and abundance in your body, in your energy field, in your perspectives, in your thoughts, in your projections, in your ambitions, in your desires, in your movement, in your breath. The unnatural states of being (control) do the exact opposite: they _stagnate_ the flow of energy, chi, and consciousness designed to move through you and out into the world as a co-creative force catalyzed by love.

Whenever we feel unsafe, part of our energy slows down because it means we're expressing from a base state of fear. Fear causes an excessive amount of contraction. When we contract and hold, we slow down and eventually shut down.

Think about your energy flow like a water hose. It should flow fast and smooth but if there's a kink in the hose, it's going to limit the flow of water. So too, if there's a kink in the body in terms of tension, it will affect the flow of energy, blood, and consciousness. To reorient this back into a natural state of being, you must not only transmute the physical tension stuck in the bones, ligaments, tendons, muscles, and fascia, you must also unravel the limitations in your own beliefs.

When we remove limiting belief systems and de-tense the body and de-stress the nervous system, we get access to expanded states of reality. Before, we may have told ourselves that "everyone can't be a millionaire. There wouldn't be enough money in the world to go around." Therefore, we find some seemingly logical reason to support our limiting belief. Yet when we expand our vision of what is possible, we can feel the truth in our own bodies and what emerges from our life as a pure reflection is the potential to experience what it will be like to experience manifesting access to intense amounts of financial resources.

When we de-tense and de-stress, we transform the low-functioning, fear-based states into high-functioning, love-based states of communicating, relating, and expressing through our breath, our movement, our energy, and our thoughts. As our tissues tense and stress and toxify, our heart is forced to pump harder and work faster. When we transmute any level of stagnation in our bodies, our brain, and our nervous systems, it's like unkinking a water hose. Suddenly, you're functioning as you were meant to be: loving, kind, compassionate, ambitious, honest, present, righteous relative to self, family, community, culture, nation, globe.

The kidneys and the heart work in conjunction to control your blood pressure. When the kidneys are stuck in a constricted state by fear, everything else in and around them is also held in a constricted state. When the heart's pumping too hard and too fast, it holds the body in a continuous state of readiness: high-alert. Until you dissolve the stress and tension and distortion that's causing you to be held in this continuous state of readiness (fight/flight/freeze), you will perceive the world as stress-inducing. Either you will choose to dismantle or generate more stress, more tension, more distortion. There is no in between. Either you are present, or you are not. If you're reading this book right now, I can pretty much guarantee that you are not. Everyone and everyone else you know has intense amounts of areas in their life where they are not present.

Those focused on inner expansion will transmute every bit of fear that is possible to transmute. In doing so, they will expand their perceptions and perspectives and will be mindful to limit the amount of negative projections they are plugging into the shared field of experience. All negative projections a person expresses into the shared field of experience gets reflected back relative to how deep and strong his or her negative projections are.

Whatever is going on in your body is going on in your life. Whatever's going on in your life is going on in your body. Most human beings are running around, using their bodies like a skateboard, as if it were simply a means of transportation. They say, "I need it to transport me to the restaurant so I can fill up my belly, or I need it to transport me to the bedroom so I can go to sleep, or I need it to transport me to the toilet so I can relieve myself completely." In this sense, it is a handy mode of transportation simply getting us from one place to the next.

The truth is, we've been given the opportunity to express and experience life like the Starship Enterprise. Yet, all around the world, we choose to limit ourselves to the experience of a skateboard. Is skateboarding fun? Yeah, of course! Yet there's no skateboard out there that's the Starship Enterprise. If you want to access your Starship Enterprise and go to places and experiences where no man has gone before, then you must focus a small amount of your attention on de-tensing, de-stressing, and detoxing. All the other beings with advanced technology on all the other planets within our Universe must be looking down at Earthlings and how limited we have become. How many studies have you seen in which they say the average human being only uses between 7 percent to 9 percent of their brain? That's because the average human being only taps into that limited amount of expression because they have accumulated excessive amounts of stress, tension, distortion, trauma, strauma, delusions, limiting beliefs, negative perspectives, and negative projections that continuously disallow us to access the higher states of functioning, thinking, relating, energizing, and emoting. We, as a race, are in a continuous state of shutdown relative to our truest potential.

That shutdown gets expressed on the inner and outer planes of our bodies. Every decade, we grow a little older, have a little less hair, our skin becomes more wrinkled, our postures become more distorted. The next decade, there's more hair gone, the gums are receding a little more. These bodies are the product of our parents' and grandparents' genetic and epigenetic predisposition. Their limitations have become our limitations, which creates a feedback loop that continues to feed into our inability to access our unique, authentic self. The more stress and tension and distortion you feed it, the more it chokes off your access to universal life force. If you continue to repeat these behaviors without the realization of these consequences, then you'll never take a real, deep look because you won't see the need to de-stress, de-tense, and de-distort. And therefore, you will die a wretched, horrible death, so the choice is yours. Would you prefer to leave the planet with ease and grace, or struggle in suffering? Either way you still have to leave the planet.

THE CHOICE IS YOURS

Fortunately, many of our behaviors do have consequences, which forces us to make decisions in response. A shy teenager lacking in confidence is probably going to have trouble establishing an interpersonal, romantic relationship. If they try approaching someone and are rejected because they're lacking confidence, that is only going to further reinforce their false beliefs about themselves and create a negative feedback loop, which must be interrupted or broken for this teenager to thrive in interpersonal, romantic relationships.

For example, the shy teenager thinks about his skillset, and because he's a good swimmer, he decides to become a lifeguard. This will also provide him with the confidence to interact with others from a position of authority and put him in contact, however peripherally, with girls. It will also provide him a source of income, which allows him to understand cause and effect at a greater level, which breeds more confidence from the inside out through the process of building inner self-esteem.

Sure enough, keeping a job, ensuring the safety of others, and trusting his own skills builds the boy's confidence, and before long, he's able to approach girls and talk with the confidence that once held him back. He has broken and interrupted the negative feedback loop. The self-esteem he established, in fact, can now bleed into all other aspects of his life.

If you're in a continual state of stress, strauma, or trauma, you'll never ever see the opportunities that are right in front of you. Even if you can see the opportunities, because of the lack of self-confidence, you will be unable to take advantage of them, so you will craft out a tiny, small life for yourself, all the while complaining, moaning, criticizing, and judging yourself and others who've taken the time to build inner and outer self-esteem. The greatest gift that we can give someone is to teach them how to access freedom from the inside out. Thinking your way into freedom is an impossibility; freedom is a sense of a feeling, and feelings don't have thoughts. The only way to access freedom is to strip away all that is unnatural from your core essence, nature, and vibration. If you're not free, you won't risk; if you don't risk, it's difficult to grow beyond your limiting beliefs and perspectives about reality. And if you don't grow, you don't discover your own unique organic ways of being and relating to any one thing—for example, love, sexuality, finances, education, religion, and spirituality. Instead, you will be inauthentic and choose to mirror what you have seen in others and what compensation patterns you developed in order to avoid punishment, rejection, humiliation, or violence from your mother and father or other primary caregivers. You will leave this planet with the majority of your core vibration plugged into the Stress Matrix. The only means of escape from the Stress Matrix that keeps you from accessing your authentic self is to de-stress, de-tense, and de-distort.

INTERRUPTING STRESS PATTERNS

The most important job of True Body Intelligence is to help you break free and return to your authentic self. To do this, we have to interrupt the stress patterns that keep you plugged into the collective Stress Matrix. The key is to be in the world, yet not of the world. I'm going to repeat this for you again: the key is to be in the world, yet not of the world. The complex stressors that humans deal with on a daily basis are by far the number one instigator that cause all of us to shift out of being inner-directed and into being outer-reactive.

Stress patterns develop unconsciously and subconsciously to cope with every situation in the easiest manageable ways possible. If every time someone went to the beach, he always turned right onto a specific boulevard, not for a compelling reason but unconsciously because he thought it was easiest, that behavior represents a low-level stress pattern. Simply because turning right would present a whole new set of attempted stressors that could either be perceived as good or bad, yet he'll never know because it's easier to continue to do the same thing, over and over and over again because, even if it's bad, we still feel safer relating from this position rather than exploring an entirely new world. Therefore, we end up underdeveloped and stuck inside the comfort of our eenie, meeny, teeny, little box. What are we left with? One choice, really. Break down the walls and interrupt our unconscious, subconscious patterns by continuing to unravel the complex stressors that keep us feeling safe in our limiting beliefs and limiting patterns of behavior through relating, emoting, thinking, and energizing.

The first job as a True Body Intelligence guide, coach, or practitioner, is to interrupt your stress patterns and establish new internal forms of communication between your inner and outer self or selves. Our job is to bring people into a relative state of physical, mental, spiritual, and emotional balance, to make sure they have the opportunity to make choices where they had no choices available to them before. Where they always turned right, they now have the realization, confidence, and inspiration to turn left.

When I initially met Roberto and learned de-tensing techniques, I found great relief from my own stress patterns, yet I needed much more than what was being provided in those moments. I was an unusual case because of SEAL training. I had put in excessive amounts of stress, tension, distortion, and physical and biochemical stress into my body through all my senses, and I needed something greater than de-tensing techniques to allow me to access the depth of who I really was meant to be from the inside out. I was left with one choice: continue to seek out, create, and develop other methods and techniques that would help me to get back to my true nature and simultaneously allow me to build inner and outer self-esteem through the process of being devoted to others in their growth, desires, wants, and needs, and their need to access their own unique authenticity.

I included all my friends in the process, and we started creating systems and techniques that did what they said and said what they did. What these systems do is allow us to move out of inorganic states of doing and into natural states of being. It creates a more harmonious way in which we relate to ourselves and others while also creating balance within all the physical, mental, emotional, and spiritual energetic bodies.

Once stress patterns are interrupted, people realize they can choose something different because their main state of being and relating has increased to a higher vibration, which increases their level of functioning on all levels. The things that were intimidating and used to shut them down now do the opposite. They are inspired to do something in a completely different way. Once they have the realization that they can get out of the hell that they're in, they show up every week and do the work and implement the strategies that we share with them. They are no longer looking for security; instead, they're discovering their own innate humanity.

This is exactly what happened to me. I was never the person who woke up thinking how I could help the world become a better place for all. I was the person that woke up thinking, "What can I do for myself? What can I accomplish that people think is valuable?" This only became clear to me once I de-stressed, de-tensed, and de-distorted that there was a deeper, more meaningful position to come from. That I could wake up each day and spend the majority of that day helping others attain inner freedom and outer peace. What could be better than that? Seventeen years later, I still feel the same way that I discovered through the process of de-stressing, de-tensing, and de-distorting.

Back then if I was going to write a book it would be, "Look

how successful I am, and these are the steps you need to take in order to be successful." It wouldn't have come from a place of, "Hey, look at how disconnected and disjointed and delusional I was. Look at all these misplaced philosophies." At the end of the day, all my "doing" brought to my life was more tension, stress, discomfort, stiffness and pain, and disconnection from myself. In order to be free, you must dismantle the stress patterns and wash them out of your system. If you get the stress out of your system, as you resolve the unresolved stress patterns dominating your internal and external systems, you will again begin to ascend back into balance and rediscover how kind, compassionate, and loving human beings can truly be underneath that stress, tension, distortion, and strauma—human beings are loving by nature. Underneath those delusions, human beings are clear. Underneath that anxiety, human beings are connected, excited, gracious, and spacious.

The root intention inside True Body Intelligence is to simplify and help you remove enough stress, enough tension, enough distortion, enough strauma, and enough trauma from the body so that you can begin to understand, feel, and relate to your real opportunity, which is to make choices relative to what you desire to experience and share it with others. If you haven't taken at least 80 percent of the stress, tension, distortion, strauma, and trauma out of your body, you have a snowball's chance in hell of finding any level of enlightenment that exists out-side of the mind. Attaining inner freedom and outer peace with the world around you will be a definite impossibility.

A TRANSFORMATIONAL PROCESS

True transformation starts with intention and moves first to observation, and then from observation into seeking comprehension. Understanding a thing isn't the same as becoming a thing. In order to become, to BE, you must transform the untransformable. Therefore, you must eliminate from your mind the false premise that just because you understand a thing, you have become the thing you understand. So, I'm going to repeat this again: just because you understand a thing does not mean you become the thing you understand. In order to become, you must take a heartfelt action. This action, this move-ment, allows the opportunity for transmutation of that which exists in a lower form and must be relative to that which you seek to become. A little force equals a little change. No force equals no change. Big force equals big change. Observation and comprehension are little forces, weak forces. Action and transmutation that lead to trans-formation are big forces, strong forces.

Transformation is an action that moves energy. To achieve a release of stress, you need to go through a pro-cess that is involved in a transformational experience.

There are four parts of this process: the emotional, the physical, the spiritual (or energetic), and the mental. To take someone through a true transformational process, all four parts must be present.

The process of true transformation goes from emotional to mental, mental to physical, and physical to energetic. Transformation takes you from being the same person in every situation to a person who has the ability to be no more and no less than what the moment is asking for. When you become stagnant in your expression of emotion, thought, energy, and movement, you become one-dimensional, a one-trick pony. It's like using a vacuum cleaner for every life situation. When it's time to cook, do you want to use your vacuum cleaner to approach the situation? No, you want to use knives, forks, pots and pans, and a stove. When it's time to travel, you don't want to use your vacuum cleaner for transportation, do you? No, you want to get on an airplane. The only time you want to use your vacuum cleaner is when it's appropriate; that's when your floors are unclean. We use vacuum cleaners to clean floors—not to fly, not to cook. Being a one-trick pony limits your breadth of experience on this third-dimensional plane of projection, reflection, generation, and manifestation.

If you choose to avoid taking the physical actions necessary to break up the energy that's holding you in that one-dimensional state, you've got no shot at becoming a free human being who can understand and take advantage of the gifts inherent within your true body's intelligence. Rather than having you be the same everywhere you go, I would rather share with you the de-stressing, de-tensing, and de-distorting techniques that will help you to realize you have the right to explore and take advantage of the opportunities that are in front of you. What might that be? The opportunity to discover and experience inner freedom and outer peace.

Regardless of where you are or what your circumstances are, if you're stuck without the opportunity to take a physical action to create transformation, you will be the same old pony everywhere you go. Your limiting beliefs will continue to castrate and constrict your ability to be fully expressed in your physical, mental, emotional, and spiritual human potential.

To explore the possibilities that are available, you must be open to observing, seeking comprehension, taking action, and transmuting that which is inorganic to your true nature. Through the processes within True Body Intelligence, it is my mission to help you make clear observations and gain comprehension, then produce actions that create change and transformation.

THE SYSTEM: TRUE BODY INTELLIGENCE

I teach my students, and now you, that I am presenting to you an opportunity to grow beyond your limitations through plugging into a system. This system is one that I built from my own understanding and experiences so that I could educate others. The system and processes within True Body Intelligence are not the thing. You are the thing and inside each of you is your own unique orientation and understanding. Your time with me should be a time to discover who you are uniquely in relationship to any one thing. Rather than mimic me, you are here to figure out your relationship to this form of work and better develop your own understanding of who you are around it.

There is a genius inside of you that knows exactly what you need; however, you have to learn a system first so that you have a framework through which you can drive your heartfelt intention. That's what I'm here to demonstrate and teach you.

Ultimately, at the end of the day, in order for you to make this system your own, you have to find your own orientation to it. You need to let God guide you on what's correct for you. I'm uncomfortable being a guru. I'm comfortable giving you my sense of what I think will be the most effective use of time, energy, resources, and the development of skills. All that I have developed so far is based on what worked for me and my own unique orientation.

If you take on my orientation as your own, then you're going to lose your self in the system, and you're going to think the system is the thing. Then your ego's going to become over-attached to the system. If I let you attach to that then you're going to hold me in a regard higher than I am. We are all simply vessels through which knowledge flows. Our opportunity as I see it is to become conscious co-creators with God as a reflection of God's love and God's light.

I understand how it is that I want to participate, I know what I want to get out of an experience, and I'm always going to make sure that I under promise and over deliver. These are qualities that work for me, but you have to find your own way. The path of one is not the way of another. Everyone has their own unique orientation and you must respect that in others and you must find your own within yourself.

I go and see the people that I choose to help me integrate because I value what they have to share. I'm paying for their time and their energy and their unique orientation to consciousness. When you come to work with me, you must understand it's the same position. You have to respect what I'm sharing with you, in the way that I'm sharing it, and I have to respect that you have your own unique timing, energy, and spirit. I have to simultaneously meet your needs while also respecting my own boundaries. But I need to respect your boundaries as well.

The first step in learning about respect is developing healthy boundaries with everyone you work with. With everyone you share space with. With everyone you have an intimate relationship with. If you respect your body, your body respects you. If you respect your light, your light's going to respect you. If you disrespect your body, your body's going to keep you from having opportunities to explore the greatest levels of experience through sensation, thought, movement, breath, and emotion.

Respect is an honoring of a person's unique orientation to any one thing. When someone comes to see me and their orientation is to Islam, any attempt of mine to have them shift over to Christianity is complete and utter nonsense. That's not my job, that's not my place. My place is to provide a safe space for this person to share what feels correct for them and support them in the direction they desire to go in regard to what it is they wish to experience. Respect is delivered to them by me by simply directing them towards setting their own unique goals and orientations by setting a clear, concise intention.

When I first started this process, I operated in a different way. I had a really cool sports car and you got to get in the passenger's seat so I could show you how amazing the world could be. Then I started to earn greater amounts of respect for myself and others, and I learned that it's incorrect for me to invite anyone into my car. It's not my job to show you the world and how it could be. My job is to get you in your car and be a passenger on your journey. I'm not here to bring you into mine. You have your orientation to truth, and I have my orientation to truth.

I'm here to simply get in your car. I don't care how rusty it is, how small it is, how uncomfortable it is, how fast it is, how slow it is; my job is to be a neutral-oriented passenger in your car during the time that we're lucky enough to have together.

I respect your intentions. I respect why your spirit is here. I have to pull back my own projections around what I think is correct or incorrect for you until you set your intention. Once you set your intention, I will get in your car and your intention will take us where we need to go. I will support you in what it is you want to experience to the best of my ability.

A Master understands that every single person in every single situation is an opportunity for growth. Rather than growing yourself, it's the opportunities that others bring to us that create personal growth through the process of co-creation. When you can recognize people for the value they add to your life in terms of the opportunities for expansion, you can become a Master in the process of life. I may have an amazing skillset, but it isn't my skills that create everlasting change. It's the presence of realizing that love, energy, life, and change all move through me, but they do not come from me.

The difference between being masterful and being skillful is this.

Let's say I'm a mechanic and you bring in a car I have never worked on. By you bringing that car to me you give me the opportunity to build a whole new level of understanding and skill. If I were masterful, I would recognize the opportunity that was being brought forth and I would reflect it back to you and acknowledge the opportunity to co-create with you, meaning I would be giving you credit for bringing a new challenge for growth to my doorstep.

The Master understands that everyone's bringing you an opportunity and that that opportunity that they're bringing to you is the thing that's growing you. It isn't *you* that's growing you, it's the opportunities that others bring to us. Giving people the recognition for the value that they're bringing, in terms of the opportunities for growth and expansion, is what makes a Master a Master. I have really amazing skills, yet it isn't my skills that create the everlasting change, it's the realization that it's the present moment that makes everything happen. The truth is, the moment is the Master. In true mastery, we give no less or no more than the moment is begging for. Love, energy, life move through us, yet they do not come from us. We are merely reflections of truth.

In my belief structure, everyone born is a genius and everyone has something of value inside of them that can shift and expand and deepen anything that already exists in this modern world. It is uncommon to see people driving around in Ford Model T's anymore unless there's a car show and they're an avid car collector or are into building Ford Model T's. Instead, there are a plethora of options on the market because so many others have taken what they learned from Ford and expanded upon that model. My hope is that my students, and now hopefully you, my reader, will take what you learn, create your own orientation to truth, and then share that mastery with others.

No man or woman is an island unto themselves. We are all in the process of co-creation. Acknowledging your brothers and sisters' contribution in each moment gives us more of an opportunity to see and feel and know the importance of brotherhood and sisterhood. The evolution of mankind shall again begin to evolve, rather than devolve. We are all parts and parcel to each and every experience lived, each action taken by all those before us, in our present day-to-day lives, and those who will be here long after we have chosen to pass from this world and rebirth back into spirit.

Part II

TRANSMUTING PHYSICAL TENSION TO REACH EMOTIONAL FREEDOM

CHAPTER 5

LET'S GET THIS TRANSFORMATION STARTED

The people who come to me are seeking guidance and education and a transmutation from their own inner limitations. These people arrive aware and vulnerable enough to admit to someone else that they have challenges, and in that moment an opportunity is presented to dismantle the quality of energy in their life that's no longer relevant to where they are choosing to go, what they want to experience, what they want to achieve, and more importantly, who it is they want to BE.

If you want to make the same depth and quality of transformation that these folks have, you're first going to need to be able to be honest with yourself. That means allowing yourself in on how you're feeling about you and others and the choices that you make and the impact others have had on you. I know, I know, I know: this is very difficult. Yet, it is what must be done. What you give is what you get. What you got is what you gave. **Co-creation.** Human beings flip strong on one side or the other; this is what I mean by that: either you're incredibly honest with yourself and not so honest with others, or you're incredibly honest with others and not so honest with yourself. Challenges either way. Your refusal to let you in on you is what is keeping you from reaching out and inviting others in to feel and sense and know your upsets and insecurities. Without the ability to be vulnerable, you're only left with the option to push down the feelings and carry on as usual. This is a recipe for experiencing greater states of disconnection, disassociation, and depersonalization. If you truly want to escape or transition out of the hell you're currently in, you have to be willing to be honest with yourself first about where you're really at in relationship to how you feel about you, your environment, and how you're being impacted on a daily basis by your choices, thoughts, feelings, energy, and emotions.

Nigerian saxophonist Fela Kuti, who produced a style of music called African Bambaataa and wrote a song called *Suffering and Smiling,* captured this human state quite well. On the outside, we wear a brave face, yet on the inside, we're suffering just beyond the false veil of what we choose to project out onto others. We are circulating in medium to deep states of emotional pain and disconnection from who we are, and the fear is gripping and holding us back from being able to take the necessary steps to build a life based on honesty, vulnerability, and transparency. It's like the line from Henry David Thoreau: we all live lives of "quiet desperation"—until we discover the value of inner honesty and begin to ask for what it is we really want from ourselves and others.

All your body wants is a little bit of connection from you. A little bit of honesty. We've been endowed with the Starship Enterprise, and 99.9 percent of all human beings are using their body like a skateboard, merely as a mode of transportation. We use our bodies in such a limited form, and once we've ignored the truth of its intelligence long enough, the body begins to fight back. Your body is tired of being ignored and abused, so the tension and stress twists you out of alignment until you begin to feel some nagging level of discomfort and stiffness in the hopes that you'll at least begin to start paying attention and hopefully reach out and seek comprehension. If you choose to ignore consciously what you're putting into your body and around you, you're bound to explode or implode at some point in the near future.

I once worked with someone who was the epitome of

quiet desperation. During our first session, she conversed with me the entire time while suffering and smiling as if she were reading off her grocery list and gave me zero indication she was experiencing any bit of discomfort. In her next session, she confessed that our bodywork session was the most painful experience of her entire life. She claimed it was more intense than giving birth. She was a two-time breast cancer survivor, she'd certainly been through the mill before, yet my work with her was the most painful experience. Again, she gave me no indication that she felt any discomfort. She had smiled through all of it, and my guess was this is what she had done through her entire life and the reason why she was dealing with breast cancer. In Chinese medicine, the internal aspect of the liver meridian moves right through the center of the breast. The liver is also the organ for the free coursing of energy or stagnation, meaning repression. Dealing with a life-altering illness is a very personal experience, and she didn't give anyone a clue that she was suffering on the inside. She kept up a good face and fooled everyone, except for her body. She learned to stuff it and stuff it and stuff it, and finally her body had said, "Enough is enough. If you're going to keep on stuffing, then it's time for you to get out of this body and leave the planet." Her body began to express signs and symptoms she could no longer ignore, and she was forced to reach out for help.

At our next session, I made her promise to tell me how she felt and what she was feeling throughout the entire process that day. As soon as she started expressing the truth of how she was feeling and decided to be outwardly honest, and gave me indications of what was going on on the inside, all the discomfort, all the stiffness, and all the pain dissolved within minutes. For the first time in her life, she was finally being inwardly honest with herself and vulnerable enough to be outwardly honest with someone else about what she felt from the inside out. What a powerful experience for her and me both.

Our human bodies crave and thrive on honesty. The body thrives on honesty. If you're not honest, if you don't let someone in on your process or your feelings, the body will say, "Fine, if you don't want to listen to me, you can keep suffering. You can keep smiling. You can keep up with the good face. And I will keep sending you signals of discomfort, stiffness, and pain, until you finally wake up and do what may be the most difficult thing for you to ever do: admit you're imperfect and in need of help."

Most human beings have an incredibly poor relationship with their bodies. They use their body like a vehicle that satisfies their cravings. They turn right if they're hungry, left if they're horny, they feed only those primitive needs and never stop to wonder why the engine is smoking or the alignment is off and the car is pulling to the left.

As humans, we are conditioned to be dishonest. We are conditioned to ignore our feelings, lest we appear weak. When we do this, however, we begin collecting greater amounts of stress, tension, distortion, and strauma than the moment before.

When I was younger, this was the way I operated. From an early age, I learned a very sophisticated strategy to survive in this world. I learned to keep things to myself and continue to make what I thought was the best of every situation. This is what I was taught: if you don't have anything nice to say, don't say anything at all; if you don't have anything positive to share, don't share anything at all; keep it all in, keep it all in. This allowed me to avoid punishment, rejection, humiliation, and violence from those who were in a position of authority over me until I was of the age where I could attend to my own needs, desires, and wants. Every time I received praise or a merit for following the rules and ignored speaking my mind about how I felt about the circumstances I was under, the dishonesty was reinforced.

Let's find a working definition for honesty and dishonesty. Inner honesty is my ability to let myself in on me. Outer honesty is my ability to let others in on me. What does that mean? To allow them to connect to how I am really feeling or allow myself to connect to how I am really feeling.

At boarding school, if I spoke my truth, I received more chores. I grew up in an environment and dynamic of imposed discipline. There was no room for speaking with honesty. There was only room for me to abide by the rules and regulations set by the institution. My house parents, teachers, and administrators in the school would rather me not speak my mind than deal with the feelings and emotions that my opinions brought up for them. If I remained quiet, stayed in line, and was a drone, and living within their tiny little box, everything was copacetic. As long as I chose to be dishonest and not let my caregivers in on how I was really feeling and being impacted, everything was A-OK. The moment I chose to be honest about how I felt about everything going on in and around me, the hammer fell hard and fast.

We live on a planet where 99.9 percent of human beings spend 80 percent of their day being completely dishonest and disconnected from who they are, and that causes them to live a life of emotional imbalance. They're doing everything they can to numb out from the feelings that they're burying, because if they stay sober, those feelings are going to bring up that which is unresolved. I've been completely sober since 2008: no sugar, no marijuana, no alcohol, no caffeine, no nicotine, no crunchy things, no sports, no stimulants, no ways of distracting myself with chemicals. Being sober keeps me present and, more importantly, honest. It gives me the opportunity to deal with the feelings and thoughts that I'm having, and not smile through the suffering. If I'm in a bad mood, you know it; if I'm in a good mood, you know it; if I'm in a great mood, you know it; if I like you, you know it; if I don't like you, you know it; if I love you, you know it. I would rather be outwardly honest about how I'm feeling and thinking than suffer a life of disconnection from myself. Altering who I am to satisfy these incessant needs from others is a trip I'm no longer willing to make. What's going on inside of me will be seen and felt on the outside. Altering who I am in order to be liked by someone else is the fastest way for me to split my personality into two. At the end of the day, it's exhausting, disappointing, and outright disingenuous. The greatest tragedy within the worldwide human condition is the loss of the authentic self.

STOP BEING LIKE EVERYONE ELSE

Most people are walking around with severe amounts of strauma and don't even know it. A working definition for strauma would be this—strauma is made up of two words: stress and trauma. Stress, once it reaches a certain level of accumulation, moves into a category all on its own. This level of stress I called "strauma." Stress that transforms into trauma.

If you walk through an airport or a mall, every person you

see over a certain age is living at 80 to 90 percent of their maximal saturation level of stress, tension, distortion, strauma, or trauma. I've worked with poor people, I've worked with rich people, I've worked with fat people, I've worked with skinny people, I've worked with extremely successful people, and I've worked with failures. Who you are in life doesn't preclude you from the impact of stress and strauma on your biology, relationships, livelihood, or success.

People have focused their lives in the direction of *doing* versus *being*. Because their focus isn't on being, they suffer alone quietly. Look no further than the percentage of the American population living on antidepressants. I guarantee you that if we put these people on the floor and start pushing into their bodies, their stiffness, discomfort, and pain levels are going to be out of this world; they will be close to their maximal saturation level in all their structural tissues, breath, energy, mood, and mental states. Yet, can it be resolved quickly? Of course. All you have to do is go into the middle of their discomfort with them and direct them to breathe relative to what it is they're feeling in that moment. If someone is able to successfully breathe relative to the amount of discomfort they're feeling and let their breath meet their true level of sensation, the discomfort, stiffness, distortion, and pain disperse within moments, and the body is restored to a neutral level of feeling, sensing, and emoting.

Why do you think alcohol, marijuana, ecstasy, caffeine, nicotine, recreational, and pharmaceutical drugs are so popular? All these substances allow a person to have a momentary reprieve from what is going on underneath. They get to check out for a few hours from the intense amounts of anxiety, frustration, agitation, irritation, anger, or depression going on underneath the surface of their skin. They're doing everything they can to attempt to feel normal. Ignoring the self-righteousness, anger, anxiety, fear, and discomfort will disallow you the opportunity to resolve, balance, integrate, and become complete again.

This is who you're surrounded by every day. Most people have no idea what it would be like to live without tension and stress, and they have no idea about the full impact of their choice to distract and ignore all the glaring signs that they're feeling deep inside. We get focused on the doing, and the rationale is to just keep doing more. The belief driving these ambitions is the reward of a gold star for being successful and winning at life. Kind of sad, isn't it? We're all so busy doing and competing, rather than cooperating and connecting.

What I want you to know is that being like everyone else is going to get you the same result as the generations before you. Do yourself a favor and go down to the local old folks' home and spend a few hours there. Ask yourself, "Is this how I want to end up?" The truth is if you keep ignoring the stress, tension, distortion, strauma, and trauma, then that's where you're headed. If you're cool with that, great! If not, then do us all a favor and take a courageous, heartfelt action by doing everything you can do de-stress, de-tense, and de-distort. Find one reason why you matter.

You can change. You can transform the discomfort and stiffness back into pleasure and flexibility. Most people I've talked to after a certain age must begin checking off the list, one by one, all the intense things they love to do with their body. Wouldn't it be amazing if you could continue to do the length of your life all the activities you love to engage in? Imagine if a fish could no longer swim or a leopard that could no longer run. In a short manner of time, they would cease to exist. Modern medicine has allowed us as a culture to extend our lives—in length, yet rarely in quality. If you love yourself and respect this body God has given you, you can begin to make different and profound choices on how you care for this beautiful, amazing vessel of love, light, energy, action, and consciousness.

Every one of the modalities within True Body Intelligence works to dissolve the stress, tension, discomfort, and stagnation. True Body Intelligence helps you to reconnect with your true self, your authentic self. When you reconnect with your true self, your intuition becomes your guiding force toward bountiful states of health and wellness.

ACHIEVING HEALTH

When we talk about health, we're talking about wellness. When we talk about fitness, we're talking about performance. The top performers are less likely to be healthy. People who seem the healthiest, as I once seemed—the extreme yogis, endurance athletes, and gym rats, professional athletes—often have the unhealthiest tissues. They have an intense amount of strauma trapped in their bodies. They're continuously putting their bodies in extreme environments. Your body can only heal and repair so much within a twenty-four-hour period. If I put more stress, tension, and distortion in my body than it can remove within a twenty-four-hour period, then my body will find it difficult to fully repair from the activities the day before. The next day I'm going to be fitter in terms of my body's ability to adapt, but it also means that structurally, systemically, and energetically, I will have accumulated a small amount, day after day, that eventually begins to compromise the health of my body, brain, and nervous system.

When I produce more obstructions than I can take out in a twenty-four-hour period, I'm lowering my power. Take somebody like Michael Jordan. At one point, his skillset was much higher than everyone else's. His ability to read the court, his timing, and his understanding of the mechanics of the game reached their pinnacle. A short time after that, however, he started going downhill fast and although his skillset was high, his body's ability to meet the skillset was low. He couldn't jump as high, move as quickly, see as clearly, or analyze as fast. He could no longer perform at the level he used to in his prime years. The question is why? The answer is simple: he accumulated more stress, tension, and distortion than he could dissolve within a twenty-four-hour period. Day after day, the accumulation of these stressors compromised his functions.

What was the problem? He had spent a lifetime of putting stress, tension, and distortion into his body at a rate that was greater than he was removing them. He could've had a career that lasted until he was in his late forties. Even in his mid-forties, he would've been better than everyone else on the court because he had the skillset and the awareness in his nervous system but he no longer had the body that could perform the action that the skillset needed to achieve his goals, dreams, or desires. The only choice left to him was to walk away from the game he loved most.

At that point, it would be fair to say that he was no longer healthy. He was fit but he was no longer structurally sound, emotionally grounded, mentally awake, or energetically wealthy. Energetic health and intelligence means being able to perform at the maximum potential that meets one's skillset. If you're no longer able to do that, it means your health and wellness presides underneath your skill.

When I began working with people, the people who experienced the most pain were lifelong yogis and yoga instructors. They had more discomfort, tension, and stress than other niches I worked with. Second were professional athletes. Extreme performers, such as skateboarders and motocross bikers constituted a third tier of people dealing with tension, discomfort, and stress. Want to know who had the least amount of tension and stress? You got it: couch potatoes.

After working on so many people, I began to understand the demographics better. Yogis tend to be weak and overstretched. Professional athletes are the opposite; rather than being weak and overstretched, they're strong and tense. When you're strong and tense, bones are required to move around muscles, rather than muscles to move around bones. What's in between those bones? Ligaments and tendons, which then get overstretched. Sure enough, a season or career-ending injury is right around the corner. Professional athletes, such as football, baseball, and hockey players, experience a lot of injuries on the job, particularly at the joint level, because of the sheer amount of force they generate in these movements. The majority of them are structurally and energetically unsound. Their bodies are lean; they have loads of muscle and can run fast, but that is not an indication of health or wellness. That's an indication of fitness. Just because you're fit doesn't mean you're healthy. Let me repeat that again: just because you're fit doesn't mean you're healthy. In fact, I think you need to hear that one more time. Just because you're fit doesn't mean you're healthy. Or well, for that matter.

The key in this process, as it relates to the work that I do, is to understand which demographic you're in. If you're the over-stretched and weak yogi, my role is to help you put healthy tension back into your body so you can again become structurally sound. When I've worked on high-level people in the yoga community, sometimes when I give them this information, they literally want to leave in the middle of the session. I never hear back from them again because it's such a blow to their ego to find out that of all the demographics to be in, in terms of tissue health, they're structurally the most unhealthy. Truth is, they can't even handle the truth. Their ego has become attached to this idea of what health and wellness is, and the second your ego becomes attached to an idea, you end up losing yourself in the process.

To be healthy and well you need a proper strength-to-stretch ratio. When I push into your structural tissues, there should be suppleness in there rather than intense amounts of uncomfortable tension. If there are intense amounts of uncomfortable tension, that's an indication that there is a major problem ensuing underneath.

If you're the athlete who's excessively strong with an intense amount of tension, my role is to help you dissolve the excessive tension out of your body, so you move back into structural balance. If you're an extreme athlete, then I must remove the intense amount of stress, tension, and distortion in your body to help you again find balance. People who do a lot of running and biking usually think that they're healthy. Yet if you got into their body, you'd find out that they're holding more tension and stress than most other people on the planet.

If you're the couch potato who's weak and tense, all I have to do is help you strengthen your body. Your muscles can only do six things: active concentric, isometric, and eccentric contractions and passive concentric, isometric, and eccentric contractions. Strengthening involves concentric contractions, gathering involves isometric contractions, and removing involves eccentric contractions. Each one of these movements does something uniquely specific.

Combining active and passive with concentric, isometric, and eccentric contractions give us broad categories of practitioners who primarily work within these ways:

- Concentric: It's about strength
  - Active: Athletes
  - Passive: Those doing house chores
- Isometric: It's about gathering
  - Active: Pilates practitioners
  - Passive: Coach potatoes
- Eccentric: It's about stretching
  - Active: Resistance stretchers
  - Passive: Yoga practitioners

Each person within these demographics spends the majority of their energy, effort, and resources engaged in one of these types of contractions. The oversight they have is in leaving out of their growth process the other two types of contractions which causes their bodies to enter into a state of imbalance that will eventually lead to chronic discomfort, increased amounts of stress, and more tension.

FINDING BALANCE THROUGH TRUE BODY INTELLIGENCE

I once worked with a woman who was a two-time cancer survivor. When she came in, she was emaciated, and her hair was thinning. When I looked at her, my intuitive body said to me, "This woman is too fragile to engage in the level of work that you do. She won't be able to handle the work."

I asked my intuitive body, "What do you want me to do?" It said, "Do you remember when Roberto walked on the front of your thighs?" I said, "Yes." It said, "I want you to do that all over her body." I said, "OK."

In my mind, I had already generated a plan of what I was going to do with her. My intuition was so loud and strong, it said, "I need you to abandon your mind, and I need you to follow my instructions." I said, "OK."

I'm an analytical thinker. I break things down and put them back together. It's simple for me. I'm really good at synthesizing information. I innately see the synchronicities and inner connections between all things. I understand how to break large tasks down into simple steps. I can come up with a plan in my head within about three or four seconds, yet analysis occurs in the mental world while physical integration takes place in the physical world. What was being asked of me was to abandon my own world to work on relating with other human beings. I had to put my mind aside and trust my heart. Then the aha moment hit me: to know without knowing is the highest form of intelligence.

Now, from that moment forward, when someone would

come in to see me, I let their intuition drive the session. I get them to set an intention regarding what they want to experience, and then we're off and running. They're driving the car, and I'm the passenger.

My job is to put the other person in the empowered position and let their energy, intuition, and desire drive the direction of the session. It's not about me nor is it about my process. On the contrary, it is all about the other person and my service is to their intention. You are now that person.

I am going to walk you through the five modalities I use to help people de-stress, de-tense, and de-distort. These five modalities consist of *ma xing*, Body of Light, ICE-centric strength, BESTS, and *Sha-King*.

Initially, when working with someone, we usually end up starting with some level of physical practice, unless they're in need of something else first. I start by helping them de-stress and de-tense all their tissues and reorganize the inner and outer rotation of their bone relationships. Assuming the person doesn't have back pain, I may start out walking on the back of their thighs, stripping the tension and stress out of their hamstrings. In Chinese meridian theory, the urinary bladder channel is considered to be the master channel, and it has access to every aspect of a human being, both physical and meta-physical, meaning their systemic organs, fluids, and tissues, and their spiritual energy, emotional intelligence, and their mind and brain as it relates to expressed behavior and thought.

Many times, we begin working on the master channel in the first session because it provides the greatest opportunity to generate lifelong impact. I can access 30 to 40 percent of the emotional tension and stress someone has accumulated over the course of their life and strip down the levels of anxiety and emotional disconnection they feel daily, not only with themselves, but also with others. With a combination of rhythm, pressure, and breathing that matches the actual level of sensation they're feeling, once the breath, meaning the emotions, match the true level of sensation happening in the physical body, all the stored emotion trapped in the cells that were catalyzed by fright, fear, anger, rage, hate, anxiety, and self-righteousness will dissolve within minutes. The goal of this session is to begin to bring them back to a state of emotional balance through de-stressing the master channel and all its associated tissues and produce soft, easygoing emotional waves in which the highs aren't quite as high and the lows aren't so low. They'll begin to feel and express the feelings afforded while moving through the world as a low-arching wave of emotional energy and excitement.

The first method I use to engage the Master Channel

is *Ma Xing,* which is translated from Chinese as "horse stomping." The purpose of *Ma Xing* is to transform the stagnated energy that is disrupting a consistent flow of *xue* (blood) and *qi* (energy) to all parts of the body.

1. MA XING

Ma Xing quickly allows me to see whether a person is the type of person that puts on a good face or is authentic in their expressions of their emotions and their feelings. If someone says their discomfort level is an eight out of ten, but they're breathing quietly like a church mouse wanting to avoid the church cat, I immediately understand that this person has a very difficult time letting other people in on them as it relates to their feelings and how they're being impacted by themselves and others, which speaks back to what we discussed earlier about inner and outer honesty.

Someone who's quite buried inside doesn't want anyone else to see them suffer or, worse yet, is applying the good face and doing to avoid punishment, rejection, humiliation, or violence. These patterns are established in childhood, and though they were useful strategies to apply to avoid these negative reactions, their best friend has now become their worst enemy. If you're an adult still putting on the good face while suffering underneath, you're left disconnected and alone. People can interact with the image of you, the identity you created in child-hood, yet this keeps the authentic self from emerging into being. This leaves you with stuffing, compartmentalization, and stoicism as substitutes for feeling safe emotionally. Quite sad, isn't it? These strategies will eventually lead to more stress, tension, and distorted behavior. Tension will begin to influence structure and leave you with a body riddled with some level of discomfort, stiffness, disconnection, and continuous states of frustration, agitation, and irritation.

The body always tells the truth. *Ma Xing* allows everyone to get in touch with where they're at in terms of what they've been stuffing and compartmentalizing. Knowing is always better than not knowing. This is where knowledge becomes extremely powerful, because the knowledge is being applied. Knowledge devoid of action is no more powerful than a bowl of soup sitting on a countertop, doing nothing. Once we engage *Ma Xing*, the inner truth of your inner story gets revealed within seconds. The first step to engaging inner freedom lies inches outside the edges of the tiny, little box of comfort you've settled into. The soup can only nourish you if you're willing to pick up a spoon and introduce the warmth of these nutrients into your body. The question begs, "Do you really want to continue to be a cold bowl of soup, or are you willing to be vulnerable and expose yourself to you by finding someone who will help you begin to de-stress, de-tense, and de-distort every aspect of your physical, mental, emotional, and spiritual experience?" The more stressed and tenser and distorted you become, the less effective and present you are. There's no getting away from that truth. Do us all a favor and summon the courage necessary to allow your authentic self to emerge through de-stressing, de-tensing, and de-distorting.

If I discover someone's breathing outside of what they're feeling, I step away from their body, sit on the floor, and talk to them. I say, "Hey listen. I'm willing to bet that you keep everything to yourself, and you find it extremely difficult to let other people in on you." At that point, they're astounded by this insight. "Oh my God, how did you know that? Nobody knows that about me." It's a common theme. I help them begin to understand the good face they're putting on is helping to co-create the stress, tension, and distortion that caused them to reach out to me. Again, here we are: back to inner and outer honesty. What noble qualities. I begin to help them understand that the situation they're in is because when they're stressed, they begin to shut off their breath. In order to be free emotionally, you have to be willing to breathe relative to what you're feeling. If you're not willing to do this, the nervous system will store the stress of that experience somewhere in your body. Nerves enervate into organs, leave organs, and then go into muscles. Whatever's going on in your body goes on in your systemic world. What's going on in your biology is going on in your nervous system. To simplify: whatever is in your body is in your mind, and what is in your mind translates out into your life. You must be willing to put away the good face and begin to let others see where you're really at, energetically, emotionally, mentally, spiritually. It's the authenticity that keeps us grounded, alive, awake, and present. Inauthenticity keeps us disconnected, ungrounded, asleep, unaware, and trapped in the past or too far into the future.

There's a great book by Eckhart Tolle, *The Power of Now*, which exposes a wonderful philosophy, but if your body is riddled with stress, tension, and distortion, no matter how much you tell yourself you're present, you're no more present than the skeletons of your ancestors. If you're attempting to control your life with your mind, it's only a matter of time, no matter how proficient you are at it, until discomfort and stiffness take over some aspect of you and begin shutting you down from the inside out.

As I move up and down their legs, I ask them, "If ten were pure pain and five is neutral, what is your level of comfort or discomfort?" The average person says between 8.3 and 8.6. At 8.3 and 8.6, they are currently at 83 to 86 percent of their maximal saturation of stress, tension, and distortion in these particular tissues. My job is to get them down to neutral as fast as possible. Think about this for a second: if pain is on one extreme and pleasure is on the other with neutral in the middle, and the average person is somewhere between an 8 and a 9 in terms of discomfort, stiffness, and pain, getting to neutral is the first step. Most people wouldn't even know what to do with a life full of pleasure. Imagine being in a body where every step and movement you took felt as good as eating your favorite meal your mother used to make. I began to discover and experience this long ago as the stress, tension, and distortion willingly left my system through breath.

Now, I had to engage my body with powerful forces in order to create instantaneous, lifelong, permanent change. Looking back, it was the best use of my time, energy, passion, and resources. Here's the wonderful thing: Once I take them from an 8.6 down to neutral at 5.0, it would take them an entire lifetime to recreate that level of stress, tension, and distortion again back into their bodies. What we take out during our co-creative process stays out.

I worked on myself hardcore for seven years straight, never taking a single day off. I needed every minute of that time to recalibrate and reestablish inner and outer balance. I swung way too far to the left; I basically put myself through the energetic, emotional, and spiritual version of SEAL training, yet instead of putting stress, tension, and distortion in, I spent those seven years stripping all the stress, tension, and distortion out. Then

I took seven years off so that I could see if the work was permanent. No stretching, no fasting, no cleansing, no meditating, no massage, no *ma xing*, no acupuncture, no breathwork, nothing. Just good, old fashioned hard work, and the work worked. I devoted and dedicated every moment of every day to helping someone get out of the hell they were living in.

After my seven-year hiatus ended, I flew to New York City and called up one of my buddies, Matt Belanger. I said, "Hey, buddy, would you come down to New York City and work on me? I want to see if the changes we started fourteen years ago are still in place." He jumped at the chance, came down, and worked on me for two hours. To my happy surprise, there was no stiffness, no discomfort, and no pain anywhere in my body.

After seven years of moving, working, bending, eating, drinking, and sitting in odd positions for long periods of time, I thought I would have at least accumulated something, but there was nothing. My body felt free, open, and as spacious as it did seven years ago when I decided to take off to do the test. At that point, I knew I was ready to step forward and begin to share all the work I learned and co-created with the world. I needed to know from the inside out, "Did this work create instantaneous permanent change?" The answer was yes. Indeed, it did. At that moment, the vision became more clear. Now I could say for sure to anyone: what I help you take out stays out. Now I was free to begin again my next seven-year cycle.

The changes that come from *Ma Xing* are instantaneous, deep, and permanent. I was once working with this kid named Jake, who was a baseball pitcher in San Diego, California. His parents brought him in, and his discomfort level was a thirteen out of a ten. I brought his discomfort levels down to a three. His parents hit some financial difficulties, and he had to stop doing the sessions.

It took a year and a half for Jake's parents to come back into financial balance, and they brought him back in for another session. In between that time, Jake had started smoking, drinking, and eating tons of junk food. Still, a year and a half later, his body, brain, and nervous system was healthier than when I left it. In that time, he had treated his body terribly, yet it didn't affect him the way it would've affected most teenagers. The majority of the tension and stress was out of his tissues. When I first met Jake, he was a mess and we put him back together. Although he was exploring in new ways, his exploration didn't have the negative impact that it would have had he had a body riddled with tension and stress. The main reason it didn't have the negative impact one might imagine is because Jake was processing the external world in a different way.

The way he now related to the world and interpreted the external circumstances had vastly shifted.

I had this guy come to see me once who was an avid golf fan and gambler. When he came in for me to work on him, he said, "I'm having this pain in my heel. It's really stiff when I wake up first thing in the morning." I said, "Oh, you've got stiff heels?" So, I said, "Can you take off your socks?" When he took off his socks, his toenails looked like petrified wood. The other thing that I noticed were these big red spots all over the back of his legs, especially on the inner line.

In Chinese meridian theory, they would say that that was an excessive amount of heat trapped and stored in that channel. But I didn't know that at the time, so I just went to work as usual. All I did for him was simple. I laid him on his belly, and I started stripping out massive amounts of tension and stress. He came to see me at least once every two weeks for about six months. Once he started to get blood and energy flowing in his body again, his petrified toenails started to normalize. This is when I realized that if the outermost extremities of the body aren't getting the blood they need, it opens people up to storing massive amounts of fungi, bacteria, and viruses.

When your tissues are healthy, the blood, lymph, and electricity are flowing. If your blood, lymph, and electricity are flowing, everything in your body is going to function at a high level. In the extremities, like your head, feet, hands, fingertips, and toetips, are going to get all the nutrients they need in order to stay healthy and well. If the blood's weak and it's unable to reach the farthest extremities in your body, then intense states of dis-ease are going to ensue, and chronic symptoms are sure to follow. My advice: tissue health must be the first step you take when addressing wellness. I'm going to repeat this again: just because you're fit doesn't mean you're healthy.

BODY OF LIGHT

When I first begin a *ma xing* session, I will begin to get a sense of the other states and levels of trauma that some-one has endured. I will immediately stop working on their body and ask them if they've dealt with any type of physical or sexual stress in their past. I inform them that it's unnecessary for me to hear the details; I only want to confirm that this level of trauma had occurred in their past. If that is, in fact, the case (and it always is if I've felt it), I explain that their body is not going to allow me to go any further and it won't relax enough to receive the *ma* in *ma xing*. I then take the person to a separate room to walk them through a system I developed called Body of Light.

Body of Light is a verbal-based energetic system used to help people reintegrate and locate the energies, consciousness, and projections that keep their bodies, brains, and nervous systems out of alignment. During these types of sessions, people sit across from me and repeat, word-for-word, the directions I give them to direct the body, brain, and nervous system with specific commands. This verbal process neutralizes the negative frequencies, projections, and consciousness and frees them from the negative impacts those traumatic experiences had on them. The results are instantaneous and permanent.

There is power in words. After all those years of going to church at Milton Hershey School, one thing that stuck in my mind was John 1:1, which says, "In the beginning was the Word, and the Word was with God, and the Word was God." Could it really be that simple? We could consciously use the Word of God to dismantle and dissolve negative experiences from our past? Wow. I love how we always remember what we're meant to remember, and in my life, this was the case as it relates to John 1:1.

Words carry vibrations. They can act creatively or destructively. They can amplify your energy or diminish your ability to manifest what you want in your life. You've no doubt heard the expression "If you don't have anything nice to say, don't say anything at all." The reason for that is because what you speak, you bring into existence by creating unnecessary resistance to your ability to manifest what it is you want to experience, which moves to another old adage, "The only thing in your way is you." Your words are the key, which brings up another old adage, "Choose your words wisely." Could it be any clearer? Kind of funny, huh? Simple and profound.

If your neighbor is angry because you cut the top hedge of the bushes too low, every time you come home, you may feel uncomfortable to be in your house because of the level of upset and negative projection he is throwing at you. Externally, he doesn't say a word, and he puts on a good face, but you can sense the upset he has inside. The wonderful thing is that instead of absorbing his energy, you can tell your body to send all the negative projections he's been tossing in your direction back to him. You can instruct your body to transmute the hate and anger back into love, so you're literally transmuting his hate and sending back to him love instead. In a short amount of time, he'll stop projecting negative energy in your direction. Hence the saying, turn the other cheek. It means transmute the negative into the positive and keep moving on. Despite what we might currently be feeling, we are all endowed with an incredible power and have the capacity and capability to do and experience many amazing things. The words we choose impact the level of experience that we may have. Think negatively, get negativity. Think positively, get positivity.

In my work, I teach people how to give their body specific instructions to locate negative projections, false projections, and fear-based mechanistic structures and strategies. Then, we send those energies back to where they came from. The body then takes care of those negative characteristics all on its own. It's a forty-five to sixty-minute-long process. Once we dismantle those negative, fear-based projections that have come into us, there is no longer an attachment at the genetic and epigenetic level as it related to our parents, grandparents, or great-grandparents. We are no longer loyal to the limitations held within our expression of our genetic potential as it relates to our lineage. Women no longer have to become their mothers, and men no longer have to become their fathers. We, as individuals, get freed from the Stress Matrix.

We leverage this innate power to generate more spiritual integration by giving specific instructions to different systems in the body. When we do this, the body will locate the discordant energies, experiences, and projections and will automatically start the dismantling process.

An older woman came to see me recently, and in our initial conversation she revealed she had repeatedly been the victim of unfathomable abuse and sexual assault as a child. Before she was nineteen, several people close to her and with the duty to protect her had betrayed her in intense, life-altering ways. All this trauma was shutting down her energetic, emotional, and physical bodies.

This woman brought a friend with her when she first met with me. We sat down together, and we located where these generational miasms and survival-based energies were and sent them back to where they came from. We transmuted them back into loving kindness and compassion. Within a few days, she was contacted by three of her assaulters, who begged her for forgiveness. And she forgave them. That was the beginning of her reintegration and re-personalization process. I have seen this time and time and time again, meaning once you transform and transmute a frequency from separation consciousness back into oneness consciousness, and you send light back to the darkness, the way-showers of that darkness—those who've done wrong to you—make their way back to you, taking responsibility for what transpired and humbly begging for your forgiveness. Light disperses darkness while love transforms the untransformable. When this occurs, freedom from the stress, trauma, and strauma produced by that event is now a real possibility.

When she came in for her second session, she was ready for me to start working physically on her body. Without doing the Body of Light first, physical touch of any kind would have only made her feel and relive the stress and degradation of those traumatic experiences. The implicate order to follow for anyone who has been emotionally, physically, mentally, and energetically traumatized is to walk them through the Body of Light process first.

She had set her intention, and now I could use the other systems within True Body Intelligence to help her unravel and unwind the stress, the tension, the distortion, the trauma, the drama, the delusions, and the illusions that were keeping her from being present. Simultaneously she was now able to access a high state of emotional, physical, mental, and energetic function. All the systems within True Body Intelligence helped her change how she related with herself, with others, with food, with rest, and within all her environments, professionally and romantically. Everything is made up of energy, and all anyone needs are the codes to understand how to discreate the negative experiences that have been co-created by us all.

ICE-CENTRIC STRENGTH

In addition to *Ma Xing* and Body of Light, I also use ICE-centric strength to work on releasing the stress, tension, and distortion from all the tissues within the human form. ICE-centric strength is a system that allows you to work with someone else who can slowly beat your force and help you generate maximum amounts of change.

ICE stands for isometric, concentric, and eccentric. An

isometric contraction is a contraction where there's resistance applied with no change in the length of the muscle. A concentric contraction occurs while the muscle shortens under a load of resistance. An eccentric contraction is when a muscle lengthens under a load of resistance. When we're using ICE-centric strength, we employ all three of these types of contractions.

The sequence in all ICE-centric focused contractions is strengthen, recruit, and stretch. The purpose is to strengthen, recruit, and stretch until all available muscle fibers are accessed and firing completely. Each sequential round of contractions allows us to go deeper and deeper into the center of the muscle and fascia.

ICE-centric strength increases function and efficiency and allows you to bring anyone who's suffering from stiffness, poor posture, stagnation, and disconnection from self to gain direct access to their nature by pulling these chaotic levels of tension and stress out of their bodies.

This system allows you to get back into you. It allows you to explore your environment and figure out who you are in relationship to any one thing.

ICE-centric strength is there to create massive structural integration. Change is directly proportional to the amount of force applied. Little force, little change. Big force, big change. No force, no change. It's all relative. Einstein got it right. The theory of relativity applies to every single thing that's mechanical in the world.

Because you're creating massive change in the belly of your muscles, it also means you can create massive change in the organ where the nerve tissue comes from that feeds into that muscle.

Think about like this. Your nerves leave your spinal column and go into some aspect of either a sense organ or a systemic organ. Then, from that systemic organ, they terminate into a specific muscle. That means, the tension in the muscle is having a direct effect on the organ and the function of that organ is having a direct effect on that muscle. If you take the stress out of the belly of the muscles using maximum force, you create maximum change in the entire system because now the rotation of the bone has been impacted, and as the bones become straighter your entire being comes into greater alignment. Since you've also impacted the belly of the muscles, the muscles are longer. There's more space in the tissue which means there's a greater flow of blood, lymph, and electricity. The lights finally begin to turn on, and you can see for the first time your truest potential.

As you do the work over time, you become more efficient. As you get more efficient, you create amazing amounts of shift and change and transformation and transmutation, as well as transfiguration and re-personalization. If and when you recruit someone to work on you, you can access the maximum amount of force needed to create the maximum amount of change in your structural body. That change affects your posture, the health of your organs, your emotions, and your energetic channels, because of the removal of stagnant energy. Stagnation corrupts by trapping too much cold or heat inside of your physical, energetic, and emotional bodies. As a result of applying that maximal force and creating maximal change, your reward is returning to a greater state of balance and well-being.

By strengthening your organs, you can balance out your internal temperatures. Instead of being hot-headed, you're cool as a polar bear's toenails.

The body becomes the brain through the nervous system. The brain becomes the body through the nervous system. Whatever stressors you have in your body, you have in your brain. Whatever stressors you have in your brain, you have in your body. The body then gets signals from your environment. All those signals get filtered through your individualized Stress Matrix you've been plugged into since birth.

Those signals then get transmitted from your brain down

to your body and from your body back towards your brain. ICE-centric strength becomes an interrupt to the distortions that have been created through perception and separation from self. What creates those distortions? STRESS. Simple stressors and complex stressors. Stress precedes weakness, weakness precedes tension, tension distorts structure. Really, you only have one option: you have to take out the stress that's distorting your structure and come back into a greater state of alignment and balance.

The action potentials within ICE-centric strength allow for an increased range of motion; a decrease in stress, tension, distortion, and trauma; and better communication between the organs, muscles, and the brain. It also fosters communication between the energetic body and the emotional body, the emotional body and the mental body, the mental body and the physical body, and the physical body and the energetic body.

When you access these maximal levels of force, you quickly shift into greater states of freedom. In freedom, you realize you have the right to explore who it is you would have become had you not experienced those stressors and levels of trauma and distorted behavior that caused you to separate from self by choosing to adopt a way of being that's counter to your nature.

ICE-centric strength grants access to your authentic self through the dismantling of the distorted self by removing the stress, the weakness, the tension, and the distortion that has you stuck in an outer reactive state rather than an inner-directed alignment. The key here is to build your relationship from the crown down. In order to do that, you must recalibrate from the ground up.

The body always tells the truth. Wherever you have pain, you have distortion. Wherever you have pain, you have tension. Wherever you have pain, you have weakness. Wherever you have pain, you have stress. Regardless of where you are on that chain, ICE-centric strength allows you to downshift back into more authenticity through the removal of stress, weakness, tension, and distortion. It's a system where you can put a person in any number of positions and access maximal amounts of change through the application of maximal amounts of force.

It is often said that God helps those who help themselves. ICE-centric strength allows you to help yourself by generating maximal amounts of leverage and strength. You're giving yourself the maximum amount of help that you could ever give yourself—energetically, physically, mentally, emotionally, structurally, spiritually. You've given yourself the maximum opportunity to create potential change, self-integration, and re-personalization.

I once ran into a woman in the grocery store who was a friend of a friend. She was limping, so I asked what was wrong. She was young, no more than thirty-one years old, and her doctor had told her that she needed a hip replacement. She was headed in for surgery two days later.

That bothered me intensely, so I called up my friend Howard and I invited her over that evening. We worked on her for four hours straight. Once we activated, recruited, strengthened, and stretched, all her tissues in her lower body became supple where they were previously tense. That change expressed itself in the rotations of her bones, and there was no longer friction where there should not have been friction.

Because there was no longer friction where there should have been friction, there was no longer swelling where there shouldn't be swelling. Which means there was no longer any fluid pushing into surrounding nerve tissue, so there was no longer the feeling and sensation of discomfort and stiffness and throbbing. That, my friends, was all gone—and thank goodness it was. There is nothing worse than losing your mobility and your ability to engage fully in the activities you love to do most.

I always sing at the end of these sessions, "Another one bites the dust, another one bites the dust, *hah hah hah*, another one bites the dust." When this young lady got up from the floor, all that throbbing, all that stiffness, all that excessive sensation in her hip had vanished without a trace of what had been present in her for every single moment of the day for the previous three and a half years. Five years later I ran into her at a concert and asked her, "How's your hip?" She said she hadn't had any of the throbbing, stabbing, discomfort, and stiffness since we had last worked together. In my head, I heard that song again, "Another one bites the dust, another one bites the dust, *hah hah hah,* another one bites the dust." For me those are great moments, creating instantaneous permanent change. Some might call it magic. Me? I call it science. Remember: change is directly proportional to the amount of force applied. Little force, little change. No force, no change. Big force, big change. The process of transformation and transmutation is quite simple. To generate maximal amounts of force while accessing maximal amounts of leverage through full ranges of motion, whatever's in there that is foreign to your nature, it will dissolve, disperse, and reformat itself back into comfort, ease, and grace.

All the cathartic experiences that I've had have always come during my ICE-centric strength sessions, either receiving them or giving them to others. In 2013, a buddy of mine named Paul Layman came down from Santa Maria, California, to stay with me for the weekend, and we were doing ICE-centric strength on each other. Then

I put myself in a position where he was helping to dissolve the tension in the lower, outer edges of my shoulder muscles, which consisted of the teres major, teres minor, infraspinatus, and supraspinatus. While I was in this position, I accessed and generated a maximal amount of eccentric force.

I used a maximum amount of force, and he could barely move me through the eccentric phase of the process. I knew in this moment that he was going to co-create with me a maximum amount of change and transformation. By the time he got to the fifth repetition, I literally collapsed on the ground, face down, and began heaving and crying for four hours straight. Paul, in that moment, emotionally had no idea what to do. Yet his level of concern was comforting enough, and he did his best to hold space—a quiet open space—so I could move through this deep emotional, integrative process. I could feel my emotional body re-personalizing to who I was at my core. When all was complete, I got up, and I was never the same person ever again. I was much more present emotionally. All the excessive intensity had dissolved, and the excess elemental fire energy in my body had drained out, and emotionally I calmed down. I now had access to a softness and gentleness that felt organic to my true nature. The intensity in my words, action, movement, and attitude had shifted immediately and dramatically. Now I could be more available to meet my own emotional needs, as well as the needs of those around me.

I've been fortunate to use ICE-centric strength to go through intense, cathartic experiences that have allowed me to reintegrate back into my authentic self. So the question is, what would be inauthentic to my nature and to your nature? Fear. Anxiety. Self-righteousness. Anger. Frustration, agitation, and irritation. What would be authentic ways of expressing self? Excitement. Love. Fearlessness. Righteousness relative to self, family, community, culture, nation, globe. ICE-centric strength is a powerful, powerful, powerful system for instantaneous permanent change and transmutation. If we classified *Ma Xing* as affecting primarily tissue health, which allows for increased unencumbered flow of consciousness, blood, electricity, and lymph, we can look at ICE-centric strength as affecting structural, emotional, energetic, sexual, and thought-based health and wellness.

If you want to integrate back into your authentic self, there's nothing more effective on this planet than ICE-centric strength, simply because you can access and generate maximal force. Maximal force has the potential to create maximal change. You can meditate until you're blue in the face. You can do qigong until you pass out. You can do breathwork until you suffocate. Yet, in the end, there's no substitution for ICE-centric strength and its ability to help you reformat and recalibrate your body, your brain, and your nervous system. Let's hand you the formula and make it very simple to understand. If you understand the keys I lay out for you, you have a chance at accessing inner freedom and outer peace anytime you want. Innate generational fear creates stress. Stress generates weakness. Weakness manifests as tension. Tension produces distortion. Distortion causes separation from the authentic self. What's the most important thing here? Creating a pattern interrupt. Where does that begin? With ICE-centric strength, because it allows you to dissolve the tension creating the distortion and separation from self, while simultaneously de-stressing the structural, the systemic, and the nervous systems. This allows you to address head-on the fear that's been held within the body, the brain, and the nervous system that's inorganic to your truest nature.

Anyone who now has this knowledge and understanding has no more excuses. You can no longer sit and pretend to be ignorant. It's your fears that cause your separation from self, and now you have a way of interrupting that pattern of fear keeping you circulating in the stress that causes weakness, tension, distortion, and separation from who you have the potential to really BE.

Moving through the ICE-centric strength process is like

taking a Ford Model T from the '20s and transforming it into a brand-new Lamborghini.

The other systems of personal development currently on the market are like taking your 1920 Ford Model T and getting an oil change. If you're lucky and combine a few of these systems together, it's like refurbishing the car back to its original state. Yet, you never get to change that Ford Model T into the Lamborghini that you want underneath that hood. ICE-centric strength allows all of you to get present and purposeful and relevant to now.

ICE-centric strength allows you to transform how you operate, immediately. Your perspective and perceptive filters shift relative to what you transmute, transform, and dissolve. The beautiful thing about this system, and all the systems within True Body Intelligence, is they create amounts of change which are relative to the amount of force that you apply—your breath is a force, your movement is a force, your energy is a force, your thoughts are a force.

If we can access maximal amounts of force, we can create a maximum amount of change. Then you get an opportunity to get into an ascended state of being. What state of being will that be? Neutrality. You see things for what they are, and you deliver no more or no less than what the moment is begging for. Neutrality is different than indifference. Indifference is catalyzed by fear. Neutrality is catalyzed by loving kindness and right action and the desire to be spacious and inclusive. From a neutral state of being, you can attain and access higher and deeper and more expanded levels of inner freedom and outer peace.

You give everyone around you the spaciousness to have their own experience relative to what they want to experience, and it's an amazing feeling to be able to provide others the access to inner peace. What could be more valuable than peace of mind?

ICE-centric strength allows you to get present to who you are underneath the fear, the stress, the weakness, the tension, the distortion, and the trauma that initially created that level of separation you experience from your own authentic, unique, powerful nature.

What I hope is, after reading and engaging in this process of thought, you'll find the courage to take a heartfelt action and begin dismantling the fears, the stressors, the weakness, the tension, and the distortion that's keeping you from accessing and experiencing who you really are underneath all that stress, tension, and distortion. As you walk away from this book, all you need to remember is: find everyone and everything you can that will help you effectively de-stress, de-tense, detox, and de-distort. Who you really are is underneath that intense amount of negative conditioning. If you think for two seconds that you're going to *think* your way into freedom, that you're going to *think* your way into peace, you're going to die with that unrealized notion. OK, am I being a little sobering? Do you know why I'm being sobering? Because I care. I hope it actually sinks in: de-stress, de-tense, and de-distort on a regular basis. Get fluid, get free, get peaceful, and be happy. Don't, and you won't. Like I said in the beginning chapters, putting stress and tension and distortion in is easy. We do that every day—subconsciously, unconsciously, preconsciously, every day we do that. I promise you: that behavior will only lead to some level of dis-ease and chronic discomfort that gets your attention every day. I like to say, "Get busy living, get busy dying. Your choice."

THE BREATH

About 98 percent of people I start working with are holding their breath or breathing underneath the moment. They literally stop breathing and immediately begin straining, which is an indication of how disconnected their emotional, feeling body is from their kinesthetic or somatic body. Most people I meet are usually only present in one of the five worlds: physical, mental, emotional, spiritual, and environmental. What True Body Intelligence provides for them is an opportunity to be emotionally integrated and present by synthesizing their breath with their movement and the level of sensation they're experiencing in that present moment. In order to get the transformation and transmutation to occur, dissolving the trapped, unresolved emotions out of the physical body is a must. You have to *breathe relative to the true level of sensation that you are experiencing through feeling.*

When I am in the process of co-creating through body work, I observe first how they are breathing. After a few minutes I ask them, "What is your level of comfort or discomfort?" Ninety-eight times out of a hundred, their breath is completely disconnected to the amount of excessive sensation that they are experiencing during the process. As soon as I identify that their emotional body is lost somewhere in another state, I step away from their body, and I explain we're going to have a potentially uncomfortable conversation. First, I ask them a very basic question: "Do you realize your breath is out of sync with the true level of sensation you're experiencing?" The answer has always been yes.

I then explain how the emotional body is connected and controls the breath, and what I want them to do is bring their breathing to the true level of sensation that they are feeling. If someone's breath is at a 1, but their discomfort level is at a 7.8 out of 10, their breath and sensation are completely incongruent. And yet, this is invariably what people do, have done, and will continue to do until they realize and understand that our breath needs to match our level of stimulus we experience in all moments. I always tell them, once I discover where they're incongruent in regard to breath, sensation, and feeling, that my assumption is they're an internal processor and they love to put on a good face. If they are bothered by how you are being when they're with you, you'll never know: on the outside, they'll be smiling, thinking about lollipops and gumdrops, and on the inside, they're full of piss and vinegar. Their perception is that you need to be different than you're being; that's the truth. They do not have the balls to share with you what really has them peeved. My job is to help them be congruent and help them be internally and externally honest about what they're feeling in each moment. What it ultimately means is that this person does not feel safe when they authentically express their feeling state to the external world. By and large, they are trapped inside behind a steel curtain that becomes very difficult even for them to penetrate or discard.

If you're getting on a flight but you don't like flying, as you start walking down the jetway toward the plane, you're likely to start getting anxious. You may begin to breathe very shallow or hold your breath. But the more you hold your breath, the higher the anxiety will get. Now everyone standing in line can tell that you're stressed, creating that negative feedback loop. Your irrational fear gets wilder.

You might imagine the plane not being able to take off on time, or you worry there's going to be too much turbulence. What if the wing breaks off? You may even worry about dying. You just keep spiraling downward until you're in a full-blown fight or flight stress state that expresses itself as a panic attack. Next, you're sweating and fidgeting, and your mind keeps creating more sophisticated irrational fears.

The irrational fear that you generated is greater than the amount of breath that you're taking in. The mind is revving up the stress state, but it's not getting the air that it needs to calm down and ground. To be in emotional balance, you must breathe relative to the stress load you are feeling. This is an absolute must for anyone and everyone who engages in irrational thought and lives in anxiety.

If I put my attention on my breath and I breathe relative to what I'm feeling, that's going to dissolve the anxiety immediately. If I choose to hold my breath relative to the level of anxiety that I'm having, then what's going to happen is the anxiety is going to amplify and begin to take over my body, mind, and nervous system.

Breath is one of the ways the body can discharge the excessive amount of negative emotion that's trapped in the tissues. When you utilize the breath to synchronize with the discomfort and anxiety felt within the physical body, the excess emotions that haven't been processed effectively leave the system and immediately bring you back into a greater state of emotional, physical, mental, and energetic balance.

Our body goes through this process quite naturally. After all, crying is merely a form of breathing. It's a physically exhaustive form that allows us to immediately break the stress pattern if we are courageous enough to engage our breath at the true level of stress we feel. The same is true of making love; the more you breathe the more you feel. Let me say that again, the more you breathe, the more you feel. Let me say that one more time, the more you breathe, the more you feel.

As I'm guiding a person back into their breath, I breathe with them at the level of sensation they're experiencing. This form of breathing in front of another person can make one feel quite vulnerable. Outside of a sexual context or giving birth or during some intense athletic event, that's generally the one time you might breathe that way with someone else. What I prefer to do is match their breath. In doing so, I am not only a physical force applying pressure and rhythm, I am an energetic force. I'm breathing with them to guide them back into a safe, emotional space, which will allow the tension and stress to dissolve the moment the breath matches the true level of sensation they're experiencing. What I do is guide them up to a 7 or 8 (or whatever their number might be in terms of uncomfortable sensation; 10 being the highest and most uncomfortable, 1 being the lowest and most pleasurable). If that person gets their breath and their physical sensation integrated to absolute perfection, can you guess what happens to the discomfort, the stress, the tension, and the distortion? Within minutes, it completely evacuates. The body transforms the anxiety back into excitement, the fear back into fearlessness, the self-righteousness back into righteousness, and the anger back into love. The most exciting aspect of this process is from this moment forward, this person now, from the inside out, subconsciously and unconsciously, begins to breathe relative to what they're really feeling. By and large, this disallows them to store enormous amounts of stress and tension the way they used to before they finally learned and began to breath relative to what they were really feeling.

I worked with a woman once who had a problematic relationship with her stepmother. There's no other way to say it: she hated her stepmother. I went through my process and as I was working on her feet, she said it felt like a 20 (out of 10). I was applying the least amount of pressure you could use.

I told her she had to match the uncomfortable sensations in her feet with her breath. What she had inside was an intense rage. As I started working on that foot, and she started matching the discomfort levels with her breath, it was an incredible act of vulnerability for her. She literally brought her breath up to a 3 for the first ten minutes, and then I ratcheted her up some more, incrementally, until she finally got comfortable, and she eventually let her arms hang to the side rather than maintaining a stiff, rigid posture.

She started breathing, and as she began to breathe deeper, she began to let go. She said, "My body is heating up. It literally feels like I'm in the hottest sauna I've ever been in." She was red, and started clenching her hands and feet.

I explained that I needed her to keep breathing, and that she could tell me anything she needed to about her experience. She remained there for thirty minutes, unable to speak, breathing heavily. Then, suddenly, the heat subsided and she started to cool down. It took me about forty-five minutes to get her to come back into balance.

I sent her a text a couple days later to ask how she was doing. She said that she had just had a conversation with her stepmother for the first time in a long time.

I didn't tell her to do that. I didn't even tell her what would happen, because I never give someone that kind of information. It influences their decision-making process and corrupts my ability to do my research. But I already know what's going to happen the second they walk in the door. There's some aspect of their life that's cut off inside, and it always shows up on the outside. Whatever's going on in your body is going on in your life. Whatever's going on in your life is stored in your body. We are all hoarders of stress, tension, distortion, and delusion in that sense. Our bodies are the mirrors of our projected reality. In that sense, if we take care of them, they will reflect back to us the nourishment available in this life. We will drink, we will eat, and we will be merry, happy, kind, gracious, present, loving, vulnerable, open, communicative, and free.

TAKING CARE OF THE BODY: BESTS

BESTS stands for Bio-Energetic Self Transformational Sequences, and it's focused on transformation through strengthening the body's structural tissues in a balanced fashion, while simultaneously dismantling all the stagnation that corrupts and diminishes the power within all the energetic systems within our body. It is a movement-based system that breaks the codependent–dependent bond you see between patients and practitioners, which for me is always the most exciting aspect of what it is I do. The great thing about BESTS is that it gives you the keys to the castle so you can go inside any time you want. BESTS allows the motivated one the opportunity to engage in their personal development at the deepest levels. In this system there's no need for guru-ship, which I consider to be "guru-sh*t." As far as I am concerned, everyone is on equal footing, regardless of your level of development. Every expression of reality in this life will always be relative.

BESTS is the one modality that is similar to exercise. However, the difference between the two is that when most people exercise, their entire focus is on concentric and isometric contractions, and they simply leave out the rest and the most powerful phase of contraction, the eccentric contraction.

There are six types of contractions: passive concentric, passive isometric, passive eccentric, active eccentric, active concentric, active isometric. If you do any one of those more than you do the other ones, you automatically pull your body out of balance. Any form of exercise that you do, if it's exclusive of utilizing all three forms of contraction at maximal force then you'll reach a point of diminishing returns, and you will place your structural body in an awkward position.

BESTS-ercise is the best exercise, and the reason why is because it employs all six of these types of contractions in a balanced fashion. With BESTS-ercise you never get bored. It allows you to access your body from a balanced fashion and pull whatever part of you that's out of balance back into balance. For me it's the most complete way to exercise your body, because it allows you to access all muscles and structural tissues from every imaginable angle, plus—and more importantly—it allows you to de-stress, de-tense, and de-distort.

The reason why BESTS is so valuable is simple. When you do other forms of exercise that have a dominant contraction you lose fluidity. With BEST-ercise you remain fluid and strong.

For somebody who does Olympic weightlifting and wants to get beyond a sticking point, they might use what are called negatives when they go to the gym. They use the negatives to increase their eccentric strength, which has a direct impact on their concentric strength. The negative causes the muscles to contract maximally and lengthen simultaneously. It spreads all that tissue open, so when that person comes in the next day to do the concentric contractions, which means the tissue's shortening, they have access to more tissue fibers.

If you're not a weightlifter but prescribe mainly to isometric contractions, which is what yoga and Pilates do, that's great. It's nice to have dynamic isometric contractions. However, at the end of the day, those will never ever allow you to de-stress, de-tense, and de-distort what's trapped in the belly of the muscles. You'll be able to reach your peak, but your peak will be way below what it would be if you de-stressed, de-tensed, and de-distorted what was trapped in the belly of the muscles.

No one on this planet should be kidding themselves if they think that the workouts they do at the gym are conscious exercise. Those exercises just put tension in the body, and tension leads to more distortion and more separation, and you get so focused on your outer form rather than connected to your inner reality.

Look at all the professional athletes. They do amazing things and then one day they blow out an ACL in their knee or have major rotator cuff issues. Those injuries are simply massive amounts of stress that transformed into tension that created distortion in their structural body. If you have a distorted structural body and you plant your foot, and you push off as hard and as fast as you can, one of those ligaments, tendons, or joints will eventually become severely unstable and the body will compensate to make up for that lack of stability. Eventually, one day, one of your ligaments, tendons, joints, or muscles will get overstretched. When that happens, your career as a professional athlete is pretty much over, unless you have the determination to put healthy tension back in the body while simultaneously de-stressing, de-tensing, and de-distorting. When the structural body is distorted, you will get some level of discomfort because you'll experience excessive amounts of friction and stress where the body isn't meant to hold friction and stress, and that friction will hold swelling, and that swelling will begin to push on the surrounding nerve tissue which will eventually lead to chronic discomfort.

If you have too much stress, tension, and distortion in the body, one day you'll be skiing down a mountain, come down in an awkward position, and those ligaments will tear because of the excessive amount of distortion in your structural body, meaning your bones are rotated one degree too far out of alignment either externally or internally.

Any professional athlete that gets injured will never be the same, because all the people who work on their bodies only address the symptom. They never address what created the imbalance in the first place. So, they go to rehab and therapy and play for another year-and-a-half, and guess what happens? They get a similar injury above that joint or on the opposite side of their body because they never actually dealt with the distortion. Distortion causes athletes to separate from their bodies. If they don't correct the distortion, it's only a matter of time before they're back in with another career-ending injury.

They can do what everybody else does and keep pouring in massive amounts of stress, tension, and distortion in hopes of being more fit but they're never going to be more fluid. Fit is nice but if you're not fluid, eventually, that fitness is an impediment to your fluidity.

Let's go over this again: fear generates stress, stress creates tension, tension manifests as distortion, and distortion leads to separation from self. Fear, stress, tension, and distortion are an impediment to your fluidity, then eventually stiffness will ensue. Once that stiffness ensues, you're going to be thinking about walking away from what you're doing because your body is giving you signals that you have distortion, but you don't have the correct tools to get out of that distorted state, so you eventually have to walk away from doing the thing you love the most. From my vantage point, that's an incredibly sad state of affairs. Truth is, if Kobe Bryant, Michael Jordan, Tiger Woods actually took the time each day to remove the stress and tension that were creating the distortion in their bodies, today they would still be dominating the game they love. Yet, eventually, distortion puts everyone at the end of the bench.

You can adjust your style of playing in your game, and you can be effective, but you'll never be able to maintain the performance. You can take all the icepacks you want. At the end of the day, there's no icepack that's going to remove stress, tension, or distortion from your structural system. Only BEST-ercise, ICE-centric strength, and

Ma Xing can assist you in doing so. The wonderful thing about BEST-ercise is you get to do it in the freedom of your home or anywhere you want at any time of the day.

SHA-KING: A NEW PERSPECTIVE

The last method we employ in True Body Intelligence is Sha-King. I met a man by the name of Earl once, and Earl was a kind and generous man. He decided to invite me and a few others to meet him in New Orleans to learn about Sha-King. I went down there to learn about the movement of subtle energy and its ability to produce spontaneous transformation.

Sha-King comes from the Kalahari bush men. *Sha* means "spirit" and *king* means "pinnacle." Historically, Sha-King reigned as medicine does today. Whenever someone was in a state of dis-ease or delusion, the Kalahari bush men would incorporate Sha-King, which would allow the person to step outside their normal patterns of movement in thinking, breathing, and moving. From that new set point, they could generate a new perspective relative to all things in their life.

In that new perspective came confidence, and from that confidence came a correct action, and in that action created movement, or more awareness, and ultimately, it created a new neural pathway. When we shake, we break down our old ways of thinking, feeling, sensing, emoting, behaving, and breathing, and we open new opportunities for thinking, feeling, sensing, emoting, behaving, and breathing. These new pathways are relative to who we are now, not who we were when we were seventeen. Not who we were when we were seven. Not who we were when we were seven months old.

Sha-King is the use of random, chaotic, and uncontrolled movements. To practice you move outside of timing which allows you to make these subtle movements, which free up the constricted, over-contained, and controlled way in which you move, think, breathe, utilize, and relate to your own body.

To do this, I typically put on Fela Kuti, and begin by slowly starting to move out of syncopation, which means out of the rhythm. I observe how moving out of syncopation feels, then I begin finding comfort being outside of timing. When you first begin this practice, it definitely feels odd, but once you get the hang of it, it always surprises you.

The thing that I love about it the most, which is why I do it, is because the heart meridian terminates in the palm of the hand. When you're done with Sha-King, there's so much electromagnetic frequency coming out of the palms of your hands it's shocking. Sha-King is literally shocking.

After I shake for the duration of a song, I can easily go and put my hand above someone's heart, and they start bawling. There's so much frequency there that it moves all the stagnant emotional energy, anger, sadness, weakness, and fear that's been trapped in the heart.

During the Immersion Experience, a five-day workshop I lead, we'll always start with Sha-King. It allows people to release the things that they no longer need. It allows them to get rid of their secrets. The thing that scars us the most is the secrets. When we're hiding stuff, everybody knows—nobody's fooling anybody else. We can all feel when someone's guarded and shrouded and full of secrecy. Often, as we're shaking, people will feel free enough to blurt out the things they are ashamed of, or guilty of. It's very freeing to no longer feel the need to be held captive by the things you did and experienced before you were conscious. Once we let it out of our bodies verbally, it's gone forever, and that experience no longer has any leverage over us. We are again free to explore who it is we would have become had we not had that shameful or guilt-ridden experience.

Now they can get back to living and being honest with themselves and others. Dropping into inner freedom and outer peace is an impossibility without access to inner and outer honesty.

The other thing I like about the Sha-King is it's unpredictable. All the other modalities have predictable outcomes, but Sha-King does not. With Sha-King, you don't know what's going to come up, because it's going to bring up what's been buried in the subconscious aspect of self where you're in compartmentalization.

Sha-King is something I only do in a group because it's more appropriate that way. In that group environment, we're all able to be witnessed, and you have all these other auras helping to bring up what's been buried deep inside you. Subconsciously the pressure of these auras and their authenticity gives you the courage to be outwardly honest about your inward shame, about some event or circumstance where you acted in a way that was outside of your ideal projection of who it is you think you're meant to be.

All the systems in True Body Intelligence allow each person to abandon the false self and get in touch and be comfortable with their real self. The authentic self for many people is very young, because it's never been given the space to explore who it really is. It's only been fed ideals and philosophies, religions and perspectives that are counter to its actual growth and expression of self.

The systems of True Body Intelligence are focused on creating enough space in the physical body, the emotional body, the mental body, and the spiritual energetic body, so that people recognize consciously in this life their opportunities to explore who it is they are outside of their mom, dad, families, and culture's ideals.

Your confused inner child must realize it is safe. Once it knows it is safe, you must then explore your environment to figure out what works and doesn't work for you, what connects to you and doesn't connect to you. Now, for the rest of your life you'll be able to seek and explore what feels right to you without worry of other people's negative projections in who it is they think you should, could, and would be. Once you feel safe enough to explore who it is you really are underneath all your negative conditioning, your coping strategies and controlling mechanistic structures will begin to fall away. What will be left underneath that pile of confusion will be you and what will be in place will be the confidence to explore your unique orientations through all things.

Sha-King and all systems within True Body Intelligence act as a pattern interrupt and allow people to break their repetitive, limiting, and fixed patterns of thinking, feeling, defending, emoting, and perceiving.

THE POWER OF TRUE BODY INTELLIGENCE

Each one of the five systems—*Ma Xing*, Body of Light, ICE-Centric Strength, BESTS, and Sha-King—focuses on a different layer within the dense physical body and all the way out to the subtle energy fields, mental and emotional states. Once you engage one of these systems, a major internal paradigm shift will occur deep within all seven layers of the human form.

In True Body Intelligence, the focus is on helping you discover who you are from the inside out rather than the outside in. Think about this for a moment: the shell of an egg cracking from the outside in causes death, and the shell of an egg cracking from the inside out allows life to emerge. At the end of the day, if you continue to keep showing up for that change you desire, that comfort that you want back, that aspect of self who you lost, that part of your personality that is no longer present, within time, all of you reemerges from underneath the stress, the tension, the distortion, and the separation.

Knowing this information now, you can no longer pretend to be ignorant. If there was one place to spend your time, energy, and resources, the obvious place would be to use these subtractive technologies to remove the nonsense out of your body. Once it's out of your body, it's out of your life. I've experienced it. I've observed it. I've proved it again and again and again and again. I took seven years off just to make sure the work worked, because I wasn't going to write a book or create a video unless I knew what the hell I was talking about. You can trust me fully: the most important investment any human being can make in their life is in de-stressing, de-tensing, and detoxing.

More fear leads to more stress, more stress leads to more tension, more tension creates greater distortion; greater distortion leads to chronic levels of discomfort physically, mentally, emotionally, energetically, and spiritually; and the chronic discomfort leads to separation from the authentic self. What is authentic to our nature? Comfort, ease, grace, presence, love, excitement, fearlessness, and righteous behavior relative to self, family, community, culture, nation, globe. Don't kid yourself for two seconds: just because you're successful for any one thing doesn't mean you're not full of the same crap everyone else is. Trust me. I understand the delusion we're all living under from the inside out, and no one ran that game better than I did.

Find someone who can help you get this stuff out of your body. No matter where you go, no matter what relationship you're in, you take all this with you: all fear, all stress, all tension, all distortion, all separation. You take it to the bathroom. You take it to bed. You take it to the racquetball court. You take it to work. You take it to your kids. Take it to your wife when you're making love. Take it to your family for Christmas. Wherever you go, it goes with you, too.

No man or woman is an island unto themselves.

Ninety-nine point nine percent of people on this planet are in that 8.3-8.6 range of maximal saturation of fear, stress, tension, and distortion. The only way for us as a global community to live in harmony with each other is to be in harmony with ourselves first. The reason why revolutions don't work is because revolutions are focused on the outside in, not the inside out. The only revolution is the evolution of all aspects of your human, spiritual form. The only thing in the way is fear, stress, tension, distortion, and separation from the authentic self.

As long as you have tension in the body, it will corrupt your thought process. It will corrupt your emotional process, it will corrupt the movement and flow of your energy, and it will disallow your continual access to your instinctual processes. When you remain loyal to the inauthentic self, the last thing it wants you to do is explore the idea of gaining freedom, because if you start exploring it means it needs to change, reroute, rewire, evacuate, and recalibrate the entire nervous system to meet your new desire to experience freedom from the inside out. With True Body Intelligence, we give you the tools and the know-how to go out and begin exploring who it is you really are from the inside out.

The beauty of this system is what you take out stays out. What we remove stays removed. What we transform stays transformed. What we transmute stays transmuted.

Whenever we remove a foreign invader, like fear, stress, tension, distortion, and separation, from the structural body, the energetic body, the emotional body, and the mental body, it remains gone. The body then immediately moves into a greater state of homeostasis. All symptoms diminish and disappear, and the discomfort, stiffness, confusion, anxiety, self-righteousness, and fear disappear. There you are, standing tall and free of the influences of the Stress Matrix that every human being you know is plugged into.

Fear, stress, tension, distortion, and separation are all silent killers. What do they kill? They kill your opportunity to experience freedom from the inside out and inner peace from the outside in.

You are free.

CHAPTER 6

DO IT YOURSELF

For much of my life, I have been privy to the idea of doing things myself and not relying on others in order to experience what you desire to experience. The Milton Hershey School, the boarding school I attended, was based on the merit system: what you put in, you get out. If you didn't make the extra effort, you didn't earn the extra privileges. You got a standard experience, which was pretty great. For the kids who put in the extra bit of effort, they lived a very different experience compared to most.

When I attended SEAL training, it was the same way: you work hard and you benefit to that degree. As a SEAL, you push your limits. You put out what is beyond your capacity. They help you discover how to put out an effort that's beyond what you believe is your capacity. You mentally ask more from your body than it is currently capable of delivering, and your body adapts and rises to the challenge every time.

With an upbringing that constantly rewarded hard effort, when I got out of the service and went back to college, I approached track and field with the same vigor. As a result of asking more than what my body had to give, I began to experience overuse injuries again and again. Yet my body began getting more and more clever. My discomfort would shift from my foot to my ankle to inside my lower leg, until it traveled all the way up to the left side of my neck. I was living in a lateralized state of function, completely plugged into a dominant-subdominant state. My left side was strong and pulled up tight, and my right side was unstable and weak. Everything I did was at 100 percent of my maximal effort. I overdid everything. I even applied this philosophy and idea when I was working with others. Every day, I imagined my job was to produce a miracle, to create the type of change that had never been produced on this planet. I did this with as much intensity as I could and for as long as I could for every person I've had the privilege of working with.

At that time, what I didn't realize was that the best way to an actual gold medal involves training just _under_ your capacity, then resting, relaxing, and recovering. I fell into the American way of doing things, and I paid the price big time. I accumulated intense amounts of stress, tension, and was experiencing chronic levels of distortion that led to separation. In looking back, to think all this was catalyzed by some type and level of fear was shocking. That's the challenge with believing in a false identity. Who you think you are isn't really who you are, and the overidentification with the image of who you perceive yourself to be will cause you to overgive and overdo for yourself and others until you exhaust all your vital core energy that's necessary to discover what it is you want to experience. I was stuck on the idea of doing, rather than being. Goals? Throw those in the trash. What's more important is what you're experiencing in the experience of experiencing what you desire to experience. Have fun with that one.

THE COLLECTIVE WILL

When I was in boarding school, one of the things I learned in church was that God helps those who help themselves. I took it in the literal sense and applied this wisdom as a rigid construct to everything in my life.

God helps those who help themselves. To me, that meant that the people who weren't helping themselves were not getting God's love. That caused me to live a life of what a good friend termed as "the life of a lone wolf," meaning somebody who lives in a continuous state of hyperindependence. I would never allow anyone to help me with anything. It never felt right, and it never felt good.

You see, that thought that God helps those who help themselves, I kept thinking that over and over again, and eventually it solidified itself as a limiting belief. Imagine having a friend who will do anything and everything for you, yet will never allow you to do anything for them.

I would refute or reject people who wanted to help me, which left me in relationships where I always had the leverage because I never let anyone in or do anything for me. I thought the only way to succeed was to go it alone. What I forgot at that time is that other people are also a reflection of God—we all go together, or we don't go at all. This was the concept of collective consciousness that I had yet to learn.

Individual consciousness equals mass consciousness. When you enter a collective field of energy, *you* become part of what's going into that collective field. When one human being triumphs over a challenge, we all win. When one human creates strife and despair, we all lose. The changes I make in myself impact the collective will. The changes that are made within the collective field by others impact me. It's equal and relative. No one, in this sense, is separate from the consequences of everyone else's action. We grow as a global community or we don't. *Whatever is going on in someone is going on in everyone.*

Initially, when I had this realization, it was difficult to

swallow. The more I thought about it, the more I understood you are I, and I are you. You are I, and I are you. You are I, and I are you.

Einstein's theory of relativity relates to material and light and energy. Yet what he left out was the creative formula, which is understanding mass consciousness as it relates to individual consciousness. Once you make a decision, that decision isn't only up to you, it is also up to the collective will to support your decision.

In the most recent Olympics, in Rio, the man who won the 400 meters wasn't on anyone's list to place in the top five. Yet he won the race and set a world record. That's an example of his personal will, yet there had to be the collective will in place to support his personal will. If the collective will did not comply, it didn't matter how much individual will he had. If you don't have the support of the collective will, you don't get to step onto that platform. It's not just up to you, it's up to us as a collective to choose to support you, your goals, your dreams, and your desires.

Everyone is a part of the collective will and anything anyone chooses to experience is available because the collective will allows a person to have that experience. If you want an experience, the collective may say, "We want to help you have that experience." Another time, you may want a different experience, but the collective will says, "No, you're not going to have that experience." Try as much as you may, it won't be in the cards for you. This is understood (or misunderstood) in different ways by different people.

WORKING TOGETHER AND SEPARATELY IN HARMONY

What I love about True Body Intelligence is that within the system are three subsystems in which you learn to work and help others, then there are three subsystems where we teach others to help themselves. True Body Intelligence combines collective and individual will all in one.

These systems and opportunities manifested so people could eventually take the integration process into their own hands. Initially, they must rely on others to get access to the information so they can begin the process and commitment to integrating into who they're meant to be underneath the stress, tension, distortion, separation, and fear; yet once they have the information, they are free to fish whenever they're hungry, and they can go at a pace that works for them. What I love about this process and the community of people working towards accessing inner freedom and outer peace is that once you get started and you experience real, palpable, instantaneous, permanent change, that change motivates you to become the best version of yourself.

My job is to inspire and empower you to start taking care of your own process. I want you to show up for yourself fifteen to twenty minutes a day and hold yourself accountable to your word so that you build high levels of self-esteem. People who have high levels of self-esteem choose a life characterized by love-based states of awareness, consciousness, and right action. People who have a low level of self-esteem opt for a life characterized by fear-based strategies and controlling mechanistic structures, which only further greater states of separation from the authentic self.

As far as the methods are concerned, we're all peers. My clients and students can do their own scientific research on themselves and don't have to be reliant solely on the information and experience I've gathered from my own efforts. It is very different from the relationship I once had with my teachers. If I have all the knowledge, wisdom, and necessary information, and I don't hand it over to you, your ability to grow your life is dependent upon my willingness to be generous with you. I took that aspect out of the relationship so that there is no need to play out a dependent-codependent dynamic, which happens to be present in most patient-practitioner relationships at any level within the personal development and Western medicine model.

Whenever you're in the True Body Intelligence community, the first step is creating a pattern interrupt and freeing you from the self-defeating patterns that you've been living in so you realize there's another choice available. If you don't have the awareness that there's another choice available to you, you're basically a prisoner in your own penitentiary. That penitentiary is a tiny little box you've been living in and are too scared to leave, and in some cases, it's more about collective ignorance. You simply don't have the information necessary to make real, palpable, instantaneous, permanent change in your life. To get out of it, you must break the patterns, meaning you must unscrew the screws that are holding together the walls of your box. All the systems within True Body Intelligence can help create an instantaneous pattern interrupt and help free you from the chains of limiting beliefs and help you recognize and give you access to the confidence needed to make different choices. You don't know what you don't know until you know. Now you're in the know. The question is, "Are you courageous enough to admit to yourself that there's some area of your life where you need help? Or are you going to continue to go along and pretend everything is OK?" If you are, remember, your limiting beliefs are affecting you, and they're also affecting us. If it's difficult to be courageous for yourself, do us a favor and be courageous for us. Do everything you can to de-stress, de-tense, and de-distort.

You're never going to be free if you choose to ignore the

stress, tension, and distortion stuck in the structural body or trapped within the cells, or the amount of chaotic energy and negative projection circling in and around your nervous system. You need someone to provide you with the understanding of how to get free of the self-defeating energies inside of you that keep you from being you.

In the first session of the True Body Intelligence process, I help you to identify and become aware and conscious of all the things inside you that are foreign to you. We keep working intensely within the systems, and we chip away at the blocks that have been co-created by you throughout your life and help hold you in this static state of anxiety, self-righteousness, anger, frustration, and fear. Where there is discomfort, physically, mentally, emotionally, spiritually, and energetically, there is no flow. Where there is no flow, discomfort, separation, distortion, and tension are sure to follow. By the third session, much of this will be transformed and transmuted back into comfort, ease, and grace, so that by the fourth session, I can begin teaching you how to apply these principles and techniques into your daily life. From that moment forward, you'll only have to put in a small amount of time, energy, and effort to continue to keep removing the fear, stress, tension, distortion, and trauma that you accumulated from the moment you were born and to this point in time. Imagine that: fifteen to twenty minutes a day to attain inner freedom and outer peace.

THE RIGHT SYSTEM FOR YOU

To break the fixed patterns held in your body that are keeping you from elevating your intelligence, consciousness, and awareness, you must choose a format that's honest in relationship to your instincts, intuitions, feelings, emotions, desires, and intentions.

In True Body Intelligence, we have systems set up for every aspect of the person who has been disintegrated mentally, physically, emotionally, spiritually, energetically, financially, sexually, psychically, and environmentally. We teach people how to maintain their own sovereign alliance and personal development by addressing the dense physical body and the subtle energetic body through accessing these five systems.

Each one of these systems is held within your own bio-intelligent organism, where your SOUL resides. Your body has its own unique keys and its own unique way of unlocking itself. You can't simply go to the gym and pump out that negativity with weights, nor can you go to a yoga class to stretch it out of you.

Meditation will never be a substitute for Sha-King. Sha-King will never be a substitute for *ma xing*. *Ma xing* will never be a substitute for BESTS. And BESTS can never be a substitute for ICE-centric Strength. *There are no substitutes*. Each of these systems has very specific ways of opening and unlocking and unraveling and unwinding the fears, stress, tension, and distortion that you've accumulated from the moment you were born and to this point in time. Just like you have to get a screwdriver to unravel the screw, bolt cutters to cut off a lock, and a hammer to put in a nail, you need the correct tools for the job.

The key to all this work is to become present with yourself. I have mastered this for my own body but I do not know what's right for your body, only you can determine the correct method for your body and that determination must come through your alignment to your creator through the setting of your own unique intentions.

THE IMMERSION EXPERIENCE: FOUR- AND FIVE- DAY WORKSHOPS

The Immersion Experience is a five-day workshop where we go deep, training sixteen hours a day, to fully understand the sources of our fears, stressors, tension, distortion, and trauma. We guide and teach you how to transmute these low-functioning fear-based states of separation back into high-functioning love-based states of thinking, relating, emoting, sensing, and perceiving. You will get the opportunity to experience the depth of all five systems. You gain comprehension of the systems and you learn how to apply them to your own life in a way that works for you. At the end of the day, *you* become the product. In True Body Intelligence, we help build noble citizens with the ability to show up, be present, honest, authentic, and impactful, without the "guru element." We are all peers in this collective mind, collective will, and collective soul. None is above, and none is below.

I'm less interested in teaching a skillset, and more interested in providing the space for people to discover who they are authentically. All aspects of your intelligence, awareness, and consciousness will increase, and you will begin to realize that you have choice where earlier there weren't choices available to you. My favorite of all is that you will begin to know from the inside out that you have the choice to participate or not participate in every level of your life that isn't working for you or is out of alignment with your own personal set of ethics, values, morals, and principles. Ultimately, you'll be more grounded, confident, excited, loving, kind, and righteous relative to yourself, your family, your community, your culture, your nation, and your planet.

CONCLUSION

RELEASE, TRANSFORM, LIBERATE: FREE FOR LIFE

The first step to liberation is education through observation. True Body Intelligence helps you make the observations and speak to someone who can help you comprehend how you got from A to Z. Through that level of understanding, you are likely to have an emotional liberation that involves some form of crying, laughing, anger, frustration, and myriad other feelings that will pass through your system like water. This aspect of the process is really the first step. Without clear observation and deep comprehension, taking the correct action is an impossibility.

Imagine a young man is battling alcoholism and decides

to take the first step to change his life. He meets with a psychotherapist who helps him process his observations so that he can comprehend how he got on the path of alcoholism. Once he has comprehended that, he can start on the path of forgiveness—forgiving himself and whoever else may have been involved. This is primarily a mental and emotional process, yet to transmute that which is in him that is not him he must be involved in a process that allows him to engage and access the parts of the body where this information, traumatic experiences, stress, tension, and fears are being held. If he avoids going into the body to create some level of true transformation, then he'll be stuck where everyone else is, and he'll be trapped in the world of observation and comprehension. Just because he understands a thing does not mean he becomes or ascends above the thing he understands.

While the external mental and emotional process begins the path to transformation, the physical and energetic process is what allows for instantaneous, permanent change. When there is no physical action, the energy of alcoholism remains in the body. This man may now *understand* what is happening in his body, but that doesn't mean any bit of it has transformed out of his body. The wonderful thing about the step he's taken is that mentally he may no longer harbor the anger that caused him to defeat himself. His transformation in relationship to alcoholism will be slight. He may be free of the mental anguish, yet in a true transformational experience, all four worlds are involved: the physical, the mental, the emotional, and the spiritual.

Until you transform the fears that manifest as stress and generate tension that creates distortion and separation from self, your body, brain, and nervous system will still be a slave to that expression of low-functioning behavior and choices, whether it's alcoholism, overeating, over- or under-exercising, lying, stealing, cheating, anorexia, low back pain, headaches, menstrual discomfort, or cancer. There's no getting away from this simple yet profound truth: whatever is in your body is in your life. Whatever is in your life is in your body. Attempting to go into your life to shift what's happening in your body is a slow, slow, slow, *slow* path; it is impossible to control your external environment, regardless of how obsessive or fixated you become. The only real leverage anyone has is in transmuting, transforming, changing, removing, dismantling, and unraveling out of our body that which is foreign to our form. Your posture is already telling everyone everything about you. Every bit of malalignment is being held in a fixed state by the fears, stressors, tension, and distortion coursing in, out, and around you every day.

To take an action, you have to physically move. It requires the body to be involved in the process. If the body isn't present, there are no actions being taken. When we teach you the bioenergetics self-transformational sequences, we also teach you Sha-King and the Body of Light. The purpose is to get your body in motion. A body at rest stays at rest. A body in motion stays in motion. Getting a body at rest back in motion requires a force that's greater than the force holding it at rest. Once we use these organic, powerful forces inside of us to make these mechanical changes within our body, brain, and nervous system, then that energy that's been sitting at rest now begins flowing in motion. It can't be stopped. When those old irrelevant, chaotic energies transform in the body, they transmute low vibrational fear-based frequencies to high vibrational love-based frequencies and allow you to express authentically who you are in relationship to whatever it is you're choosing to experience.

If you don't have the ability to authentically express your wants, desires, and needs, they'll never come to fruition. That means you'll spend a lifetime sacrificing yourself to meet the needs of others. You will crave that recognition from your mom and dad to prove that you are worthy. You will crave recognition from others, and you will put on masks so that you don't have to be vulnerable. The fact is, you already have worth. You don't need anyone else to determine whether you have value: you already have value. The more you choose to show up for you, the greater your value becomes.

True integration begins when we become v
Vulnerability is where we allow ourselves
our desires in the most authentic ways. When w̖
in stress, tension, distortion, trauma, and strauma, our
energetic body becomes stagnant, and emotionally we
begin to close off to the world. When we are vulnerable,
we are able to receive the authenticity of others without
the need to control how they are being in any way, shape,
or form. If you move through the world and you're not
in the receptive mode—meaning you lack the ability to
receive love, consciousness, awareness, insight, help,
and understanding from other human beings—you're
left alone, an island unto yourself. You can be among a
crowd of the most amazing people, but you will feel like
a lone wolf living in separation.

When you open yourself up to receive, you become consciously reconnected to the collective. You become open
to the true you. You get a new choice point. Instead of
always going left, you now have the ability and confidence to turn right. This begins an exploratory phase of
life, of discovering who it is you are in this phase of life,
and involves re-parenting oneself and asking some tough
questions: who am I in relation to food? to sexuality? to
religion? to education? to emotion? to my community?
to my finances?

Once you begin to engage in this process, you start to

redesign your life from the inside out and distress is no longer a catalyzer for your success. You begin to act, emote, feel, think, and be in all the ways in which you want to be. You're no longer held in by obligation and fantasy; you're completely OK with reality. Seventeen years ago, if one of my brothers had asked me if I'd be at his daughter's wedding in June, I'd have said, "Of course!" no matter what kind of burden that might have meant for me at that time. Today, if asked the same question from the same people, I'm comfortable saying that I need to wait and see what I have planned at that time. This gives me the time to assess whether or not going to the wedding is the correct action for me.

Most people would say, "Oh my god, this is your brother's daughter. Are you kidding me? You're not going to show up for the wedding? She only gets married once in her life."

While that may be true, I'm a free human being. I get to choose to participate in my life in the ways in which I want: right, wrong, good, bad, correct, and incorrect are not part of my thought process. Doing something out of co-dependency, dependency, fear, rejection, humiliation, punishment, guilt, or shame is the worst form of slavery. And that's how the rest of the world is operating every day. Whereas, if I genuinely want to go because I want to support her, that's different: I'm doing it out of my own volition as opposed to out of obligation. Most human beings do things out of obligation, creating more stress, more tension, and more distortion. All this is catalyzed by fear and an avoidance of rejection, humiliation, punishment, guilt, shame, or violence. If you live in this way, you're simply acting to protect your outer self-esteem.

Outer self-esteem and recognition are the things you do with and for others. Inner self-esteem is something you do with and for yourself. We've all been brainwashed to believe that selflessness is a virtuous quality and selfishness is a vice. The reality is selflessness is the same as selfishness and vice versa: they're two extremes of the same frequency. Obligation disallows us to be clear on what is correct for each of us in that moment of choice; obligation is a shackle.

You need to have portions of your life in which you ought to be selfish and put your needs first. Once you've tended to those needs and built your inner self-esteem, then you have something to offer others. Otherwise, you're doing the same old thing and giving from an empty place: looking for outer recognition that you have value is like getting a gold star that shows you're winning at life. In reality, a gold star is just a sticker on a piece of paper. The only win that you can ever receive in this world is discovering who you are. *You're only winning if you're being you.* If you're not being you, you're losing. Success can only be defined as one's ability to be authentically expressed in the world. Any achievement you gain while not being you is a failure. There is no way around this.

When you do things for yourself, you build inner self-esteem. If you commit to the process and don't break from it, your self-esteem will rise. By continuing the process, you create a natural flow in your life that is all done by you: *your* body, *your* mind, *your* energy, *your* breath, *your* movement, *your* consciousness, and *your* choice.

My goal for people is to help them meet themselves. Once people meet themselves, they're free to explore every aspect of their environment in which they choose to know themselves. Their pain, anxiety, confusion, anger, frustration, agitation, self-righteousness, and fear disappear at varying levels and degrees relative to how engaged they are in the process of True Transformation. All this leads to outer peace with everything around you. No need for control, no need to continue reengaging ideas, feelings, and expressions of emotion that are irrelevant to who you are today.

Once you're a free human being, you're no longer plugged into the Stress Matrix everyone else is operating in. When everyone else goes left, you only go left if it feels right for you, if it makes sense to you, if it's in alignment with who you are. You only go right if it feels right for you, if it makes sense to you, if it's in alignment with who you are. You're not going right because you're rebelling against the system, you're going right because that's what feels good for you, and you're willing to take all the risk necessary to experience who it is you are in that moment. It has nothing to do with the externality; it has everything to do with the internal choice. You realize that you have the right to make choices about what you want to experience, while simultaneously understanding clearly you have the right to participate or no longer participate in things that no longer feel correct to you. You are no longer a slave to obligation. That alone is worth the effort.

The discomfort that you had in your body, heart, emotions, or mind that's been torturing you energetically, physically, mentally or emotionally is gone. You will walk around in a joyous state because you realize you have the freedom to choose the life you want from the inside out without the fear or worry of approval from the outside in. You no longer have to be loyal to the false projections of who you think you are or what you think you should be. Your nervous system will re-calibrate to a new set point in relationship to gravity, space, time, and consciousness.

You will now be free. Free to explore the depth and truth of who it is you have always been and are meant to be. Free for life.

MAJOR
TAKEAWAYS

Whatever's going on in your body is going on in your life. Whatever's going on in your life is stored in your body.

Your success doesn't mean you've escaped the bullsh*t everyone else has.

The more you breathe, the more you feel.

The key is to be in the world, yet not of the world.

Understanding a thing does not mean you become the thing you understand.

Just because you're fit doesn't mean you're healthy.

The body will keep sending you signals of discomfort, stiffness, and pain, until you finally wake up and do what may be the most difficult thing for you to ever do: admit you're imperfect and in need of help.

That "me" was under the armor, and my armor was so strong that people couldn't reach me and feel who I really was.

Who are you? If you don't know who you are, you don't know why you're doing what it is you're doing. If you don't know why you're doing what you're doing, you can't question your motivations.

People's perception of me was based on how much tension I was holding.

The preferred form of relating was through sarcasm and stoicism. Now I was surrounded by people whose primary way of relating was through humor and vulnerability.

There was so much change and the only thing I did was remove stress, tension, and distortion.

Unsolicited feedback I got from others confirmed how important the changes I was making really were.

The truth is there's no substitute. Either you're stressed,

tense, and distorted, or you're not. If you are, you need to pull down the wall right now, get vulnerable, and ask for help.

Keep lobbing in more stress, keep accumulating more tension and more distortion, and you know what you're going to get? You're going to get further, further, and further away from yourself and you're going to be operating at low functioning behaviors (doing) versus high functioning behaviors (being). What it really comes down to is this: do you want to do, or do you want to be? Doing is a prison sentence, and the only escape is seeking freedom from the inside out.

There comes a day where every boy looks at his father and decides he's going to do things his own way. It took me two years and three months to mature to that state of readiness and have the realization that it was time to do my own thing and discover the truths within truth for myself.

It took an extremely courageous woman to get me to understand that magic is what happens in the gray areas of life.

That truth would eventually become my North Star, my mission, my motivating force in life, which I call True Body Intelligence.

High levels of intelligence enable us to move forward as a culture and a race. If we lack understanding of each physical, mental, emotional, spiritual, energetic, and sexual aspect, it becomes impossible for us to navigate the challenges coming to us next.

The greatest gift in life is people that care enough to tell us how we're impacting them.

This is why it's best to surround yourself with people who care enough to tell you the things you don't want to hear.

True Body Intelligence breaks the co-dependent/dependent patient-practitioner dynamic that disempowers the patient and practitioner.

We underpromised and overdelivered.

Listen first. Gather the data, and respond and initiate appropriately.

If you choose to become a parrot, what you give up is the opportunity to discover who you are.

I needed to find my own orientation in order to be effective in the world; I had to take ownership of who I was becoming.

True Body Intelligence is an opportunity to change and transform that which is inevitable. There will never be any more or any less energy in your body, it only matters whether or not you have access to it.

When I understand the why behind someone's motivation, I can make the personal choice of whether or not to participate.

Intelligence is one's ability to manipulate their environment to produce the result that they want to experience.

"Where there is pain there is no flow; where there is no flow, pain is sure to follow."

The experience of freedom is really meant for those who truly desire to experience human potential at its greatest level.

You have to focus on developing your physical, mental, emotional, environmental, and spiritual intelligence. You must focus a bit of your time, energy, and resources on detoxification. You need to focus a bit of your time and energy on structural integration. You need to focus a bit of your time and energy on meditation. You should focus a bit of your energy on psychological and emotional development. Lastly, you need to focus an intense amount of time, energy, and resources on de-stressing and de-tensing if you're ever going to reach even close to your individual human potential that lies within your own innate genius.

Vulnerability is the ascended quality because it shifts you emotionally and physically into the receptive mode.

True Body Intelligence is about creating a pattern interrupt and breaking down the density and dismantling the stress that keeps those walls and boxes fixed, unmovable, and rigid. When you finally decide to break down those walls, you suddenly have the experience, for the first time in your life, of being.

Doing suddenly seems ridiculous and nonsensical. Being has great inner value. Doing has some outer value. It's more important to Be open-minded than it is to do research. It's more important to Be in a state of inner freedom than it is to go on vacation. It's more important to Be in a state of peacefulness than it is to sacrifice yourself to maintain relationships with others.

If you're willing to move through your fears, be completely present, and take the correct action necessary to achieve what it is you want to experience, you will find that life is quite rewarding. If you do the inverse, you will find life to be quite defeating. And in so doing you will discover that whatever fears you're unwilling to move through actually capture you and steal your opportunity to connect to your authentic self.

The greatest gift that we can give someone is to teach them how to access freedom from the inside out.

If you're not free, you won't risk; if you don't risk, it's difficult to grow beyond your limiting beliefs and perspectives about reality.

The most important job of True Body Intelligence is to help you break free and return to your authentic self.

The first job as a True Body Intelligence guide, coach, or practitioner, is to interrupt your stress patterns and establish new internal forms of communication between your inner and outer self or selves.

The system and processes within True Body Intelligence are not the thing. You are the thing and inside each of you is your own unique orientation and understanding.

Our opportunity as I see it is to become conscious co-creators with God as a reflection of God's love and God's light.

A Master understands that every single person in every single situation is an opportunity for growth.

What you give is what you get. What you got is what you gave. Co-creation.

If you truly want to escape or transition out of the hell you're currently in, you have to be willing to be honest with yourself first about where you're really at in relationship to how you feel about you, your environment, and how you're being impacted on a daily basis by your choices, thoughts, feelings, energy, and emotions.

Altering who I am to satisfy these incessant needs from others is a trip I'm no longer willing to make.

If someone is able to successfully breathe relative to the amount of discomfort they're feeling and let their breath meet their true level of sensation, the discomfort, stiffness, toxicity, and pain disperse within moments, and the body is restored to a neutral level of feeling, sensing, emoting, and being.

We get focused on the doing, and the rationale is to just keep doing more. The belief driving these ambitions is the reward of a gold star for being successful and winning at life. Kind of sad, isn't it? We're all so busy doing and competing, rather than cooperating and connecting.

Energetic health and intelligence means being able to perform at the maximum potential that meets one's skillset. If you're no longer able to do that, it means your health and wellness presides underneath your skill.

Strengthening involves concentric contractions, gathering involves isometric contractions, and removing involves eccentric contractions. Each one of these movements does something uniquely specific.

What's going on in your biology is going on in your nervous system. Whatever is going on in your nervous system is going on in your mind. To simplify, whatever is in your body is in your mind, and whatever is in your mind translates out into your life.

The key here is to build your relationship from the crown down. In order to do that, you must recalibrate from the ground up.

Remember: change is directly proportional to the amount of force applied. Little force, little change. No force, no change. Big force, big change. *(Hint, hint!)*

What's the most important thing here? Creating a pattern interrupt.

As you walk away from this book, all you need to remember is: find everyone and everything you can that will help you effectively de-stress, de-tense, and de-distort.

The reason why revolutions don't work is because revolutions are focused on the outside in, not the inside out.

What's more important is what you're experiencing in the experience of experiencing the experience. Have fun, and then let it go.

People who have high levels of self-esteem choose a life characterized by love-based states of awareness, consciousness, and right action. Those who have low self-esteem choose a life characterized by fear-based states of awareness, consciousness, and inaction.

The first step to liberation is education through observation that leads to comprehension.

When there is no physical action, the energy of alcoholism remains in the body. This man may now understand what is happening in his body but that doesn't mean any bit of it has transformed out of his body.

To take an action, you have to physically move.

True integration begins when we become vulnerable.

ABOUT THE AUTHOR

CHRISTOPHER LEE MAHER is a former Navy SEAL who endured physical stress and trauma as a result of his training and conditioning during and after his military career, then exacerbated that damage by attempting to fulfill his Olympic dream. He studied Traditional Chinese Medical Practices at the Pacific College of Oriental Medicine and Yo San University. He has also continued his studies at The Universal Healing Tao System, and is a student of Grand Master Mantak Chia at the Universal Tao Master School in Chiang Mai, Thailand. He is currently pursuing his master's and doctorate degrees in Traditional Chinese Medicine.

He has taught himself how to free his body, brain, and nervous system from dis-ease by distinguishing between the emotional, physical, mental, and spiritual aspects of being. Today, he travels the world, teaching others to find the same freedom for themselves.

Find Christopher at www.truebodyintelligence.com

Made in the USA
Columbia, SC
05 August 2022

64665440R10152